W9-AQO-499

SEVEN TRANSFORMING GIFTS OF MENOPAUSE

AN UNEXPECTED SPIRITUAL JOURNEY

CHERYL BRIDGES JOHNS

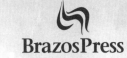

Brazos Press
a division of Baker Publishing Group
Grand Rapids, Michigan

Published by Brazos Press
a division of Baker Publishing Group
PO Box 6287, Grand Rapids, MI 49516-6287
www.brazospress.com

Printed in the United States of America

Library of Congress Cataloging-in-Publication Data
Names: Johns, Cheryl Bridges, author.
Title: Seven transforming gifts of menopause : an unexpected spiritual journey / Cheryl
    Bridges Johns.
Description: Grand Rapids, Michigan : Brazos Press, a division of Baker Publishing
    Group, [2020] | Includes bibliographical references and index.
Identifiers: LCCN 2019035660 | ISBN 9781587434396 (paperback)
Subjects: LCSH: Menopause—Religious aspects—Christianity. | Middle-aged women—
    Religious life. | Middle-aged women—Health and hygiene.
Classification: LCC RG186 .J64 2020 | DDC 618.1/75—dc23
LC record available at https://lccn.loc.gov/2019035660

Published in association with Books & Such Literary Management, www.booksandsuch.com.

20 21 22 23 24 25 26   7 6 5 4 3 2 1

In keeping with biblical principles of creation stewardship, Baker Publishing Group advocates the responsible use of our natural resources. As a member of the Green Press Initiative, our company uses recycled paper when possible. The text paper of this book is composed in part of post-consumer waste.

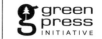

This book is dedicated
to the memory of Waneda Brownlow.

Missionary.
Teacher.
Advocate for women's rights.
A woman reborn in her fifties.

Until her last breath,
Waneda was in her heart "fifteen, a happy fifteen."

CONTENTS

PREFACE

SEVEN TRANSFORMING GIFTS OF MENOPAUSE is not meant to be an exhaustive treatment of menopause or a medical textbook. It serves as a developmental and spiritual guide, pointing out some major landmarks for your menopausal journey. Consider it the *Lonely Planet* version of menopause, taking you down some roads less traveled so that you can discover the hidden sweet spots.

Seven Transforming Gifts of Menopause is an encouraging work, designed to help you take note of the gifts in the rich ecology in the land of menopause. It is not another impossible standard for women to reach. There is no pressure to receive all the gifts. Feel free to take what you wish. Leave the rest. You may be at a place in life where you are ready for only one or two gifts. Don't worry. Years from now you can revisit the gifts, perhaps finding it possible to receive a couple more. You are free to disregard things that have little relevance to your life as you use this guide to blaze your own trail. While women face common challenges, there is no one-size-fits-all journey through menopause.

Seven Transforming Gifts of Menopause is a gentle space. I write as an older woman desiring to take you by the hand to lead you through the rough terrain toward the wonderland of menopause. Along the way, I will ask you to consider things about yourself, your past, your present, and your future. If at any time these questions become too difficult or painful, feel free to move to another section.

Seven Transforming Gifts of Menopause is designed to be a safe place where you can read, ponder, remember, pray, and cry. It provides space to express regret. It gives you permission to speak the unspoken. It provides nonjudgmental space for anger and tears. In other words, it is perfectly okay to be a hot mess while exploring this book.

Seven Transforming Gifts of Menopause is a deeply personal space. At the end of each chapter, you will find questions designed to help you reflect on your journey. These questions will assist you in probing your psyche to find healing and experience growth. They offer an opportunity for you to place your unique experiences in dialogue with the material.

Seven Transforming Gifts of Menopause is a communal space. If you so choose, you can participate in a reading/discussion group for this book. At the end of each chapter, I have provided group activities and questions designed to facilitate open and honest dialogue. You may find that traveling in the company of women will help make the menopausal journey more beneficial. It is hard to travel alone. You are more likely to make it through to the other side if others are encouraging you along your journey.

Seven Transforming Gifts of Menopause is a sacred space where you can discover a deeper, more mature relationship with God. I am writing as a Christian, but you do not have to be a Christian to benefit from this book. Women of all faith traditions are welcome along on this journey. There is no "Christian menopause" or "Jewish menopause" or "Muslim menopause," but our faith traditions color and shape the developmental tasks of menopause. Some faith traditions hold to a more traditional view of "a woman's place." For that reason, women from more conservative religions may find some sections of this book to be especially challenging. I encourage you, whatever your faith tradition, to look for opportunities to discover a deeper, more mysterious, more loving God.

Throughout this book you will discover personal stories about women. When only first names are given, I have used pseudonyms in order to protect anonymity. In many cases, I have altered the stories, changing dates and locations.

A word of warning: the journey into the land of menopause is not for the faint of heart. The gifts found in this land are not easily claimed. As you travel, people will try to convince you that the transformation you are undergoing is not for the good. They will tell you that it is selfish to desire the gifts of menopause. They will tell you that the ideas, the feelings, and the desires you are experiencing are products of your overactive hormonal system. People will suggest that the fruit you find in this wonderland is forbidden for "nice girls." These people are everywhere: communities, family systems, places of worship, and the media. You know these people well, but don't let them override the truth emerging from deep within you.

I invite you to take and read. Forge ahead into the gift-filled land of menopause. Taste the fruit. Drink from the springs. Travel all the way to the seventh gift, the gift of your courageous, adventurous self. If you make it there, you will become a person no one, including yourself, ever imagined you could be. That person lies in wait in the dragon's den.

ACKNOWLEDGMENTS

WRITING IS BOTH A SOLITARY TASK as well as a communal one. It takes a village to write a book. My village includes my husband of forty-five years, Jackie David Johns. During my rough ride through perimenopause, it was he who suggested I write a book about the experience. My daughters, Alethea and Karisa, have been a great source of joy and inspiration during the many years of writing this book. My agent, Rachelle Gardner, helped me realize that I was not alone in believing that Christian women could use some help in claiming the gifts of menopause. My editor, Robert Hosack, from our initial conversation about the book until its publication, has been a gift. Finally, my teaching assistant, Shoba Jacob, has been a steady presence and insightful editor.

INTRODUCTION

A FEW YEARS AGO, I set out on a journey into the strange and frightening land called menopause. Looking back, I realize how woefully unprepared I was for the trip. I had no map. I had not read any books that would help me on my way. No one volunteered to serve as my travel guide.

I had heard a few stories about the place to which I was going. It had a climate that could get very hot. It was hard to sleep there. It was, at times, a place of trauma and suffering. In my family, there were tales about "the crazy aunt" who, after having gone there, was never the same. There was even a frightening story of my great-aunt who bled to death in the land of menopause.

Before setting out on the journey, I tried to talk to a couple of women who had gone to the same place; perhaps they would give me some pointers. They only stared at me in stony silence as if to make it clear that I had broken some unspoken rule by asking about their sojourn.

Knowing that this quest was a fate coded in my DNA did little to curb my fears. I feared I would come out on the other side mentally damaged like those traumatized travelers many whispered about. Or maybe, like my great-aunt—the one whose face in faded photographs was the most beautiful I had ever seen—I would simply bleed to death.

In addition to not knowing what to expect, I did not know when my menopausal journey would begin. For certain, there would be no letter informing me to show up at the borderland of menopause on such and such day in such and such month. I knew there would be warning signs. So I waited for the signs.

I waited for years, until I was well past the age of fifty, with no notice of the impending trip. People began telling me that it was rare to wait so long to travel to this land. Sometimes they spoke as if I were somehow to blame for the delay. My physician wondered if I was "normal." I tried to explain the delay: "I think my mother waited a long time."

One day in my mid-fifties, I found myself standing at the borderland between my home and this new land. My time had come. The signs were certain. I had to leave the comforts of my earlier life and walk alone into the great unknown.

As soon as I set foot into the new terrain, it became clear that my fears were legitimate. I learned quickly that menopause was a place that made up its own rules. Life skills from my prior existence had no effect here. The harder I tried to adapt, the worse things became. For the first few months of the journey, I was a complete mess. I did not know how to think. I did not know how to sleep. I did not know how to live.

There should have been a warning sign at the border of this land of menopause that read, "Beware! You are about to enter a haunted landscape!" I believe such a notice would have prepared me for the ghosts of my past who, as I made my way along, rose from their graves and demanded my attention. Had there been such a sign, I might have braced myself for the appearance of the vivid images of events long forgotten. Past injustice, hurt, and shame that I once thought were buried came back with a vengeance.

Remembering caused me to become angry. I do not mean a mild annoyance but an intense, deep anger. It seemed that the more I remembered, the more I saw people for how they really were and the angrier I became. Truthfully, the remembering and the anger overcame me. I could not get over things as I once did.

The anger and the remembering brought on tears. My eyes became red from weeping. I wept over the pain, the injustice, and the unfairness in my life. I wept over my marriage. I wept over my children. I wept over the world. I wept over my anger. I wept in frustration over my inability to control my tears.

One day the bleeding started. It did not trickle out. It came in great gushes, leaving my body weak and my clothing soaked. I bled so much that I became anemic. My hair became brittle. Dark circles appeared under my tear-soaked eyes. I thought of my great-aunt. Did she die from anemia? Did her beautiful face become discolored like mine? Did she simply not wake up one morning after bleeding out?

As I went deeper into this land, I began to believe I had entered hell itself. At times, especially at night, it felt as hot as hell. It seemed the life I had once known—the one character-ized by control, accomplishment, and the ability to let things go—would never return. I feared I would always be an angry, teary, hot, and bleeding person living in this godforsaken land of menopause.

When I say "godforsaken," I mean it literally. It felt as if God had stood at the borderland of menopause and waved good-bye—leaving me to face the anger, tears, and bleeding alone. To be hon-est, at times my tears and anger were directed at God. I would not have blamed God for not wanting to be around me. My husband often looked as if he wanted to escape.

During my sojourn in this desolate wilderness, I had one re-curring fantasy. I imagined lying down and wrapping myself in a shroud. Here in the midst of the wilderness, the winds would cover me in sand, creating a silent tomb where the pain, anger, and bleeding would disappear. Strangely, this image held great comfort—so much so that it became my safe place when things became unbearable.

Then, just as I resigned myself to this hell, I began to realize that this land wasn't all that I had feared it to be. Certainly, it was a place of my undoing. But, if I was being honest, there were things in my life in need of undoing. It was a place of anger, but anger is, at times, a good thing. It was a haunted land, but on occasion, the ghosts of the past return to give us a second chance.

Yes, I was in a godforsaken place, but a God more mysterious, more open to paradox replaced the God who forsook me. My previous God was one of order, green pastures, and still waters. This God seemed to relish the fierce storms that arose without warning in the land of menopause. The God of my past seemed to stand afar, looking down on my life. The God I discovered in the midst of the wind and darkness of the godforsaken land called menopause did not stand far off, repulsed by the hot mess I had become. Instead, this God drew close, surrounding me with gentle wings. In the midst of the darkness, I then understood that my longing to be wrapped in a shroud was actually a deep desire to be wrapped in a cocoon. Hidden under the Spirit's wings, I waited to be reborn. I could sense that what was waiting to be born was good, very good.

I had reached a point where I saw the land of menopause for what it was: a special space wherein I could rewrite the story of my life. I was passing through a portal into a richer and fuller way of being in the world. I knew then that if given the opportunity

4

to turn back, I would not do so. I had found the crucible of my remaking.

What Is Menopause?

Like most women, I entered "the change" unprepared. I was well educated, living in the twenty-first century, yet no one had prepared me for what to expect during menopause. As was the experience of millions of others before me, I faced a great unknown. I knew there were drugs available should things become rough, but for the most part, I had little knowledge about what would become a significant part of my life journey. I was both unaware and fearful.

What is menopause? What happens to women's bodies during this time? Technically, menopause is the cessation of menstruation. It is the culmination of complex hormonal changes that began ten to fifteen years earlier. Often these changes are so subtle that women never notice. For instance, during our twenties, our monthly cycles probably lasted about thirty-two days. By the time we reached our mid-thirties, the length had probably decreased to twenty-eight days. This change is due to maturing follicles producing less progesterone during each cycle, shortening the period of time when the uterine lining is thickened in preparation for a fertilized egg.

As women move into their forties, the time between their periods may become erratic, ranging from twenty-one days to twenty-eight days. Eventually, the intervals begin to lengthen and menstruation stops altogether. Every woman's journey into menopause is different. Some women, such as myself, take the long route, reaching menopause in their late-fifties. Other women take the short route, reaching menopause during their mid-forties. The

average age of the onset of natural menopause in the industrial-
ized world is 51.4 years.[1]

Perimenopause

The journey into menopause begins with a transitional phase
known as perimenopause. The typical age when this transition
begins is 47.5 years. The length of the transition can be as short as
one year and as long as twelve years. The typical length of transition is 5.8 years.[2] Perimenopause is when the most dramatic brain
and hormonal changes occur in the female body. Perimenopause
begins with changes in a woman's brain chemistry caused by al-
terations in the delicate interaction between the hypothalamus,
the pituitary gland, the ovaries, and the key hormones that are
produced in these areas. During perimenopause, the body attempts to navigate the upheaval of the delicate balance of estrogen,
progesterone, and androgens.

As a woman's body struggles to adapt to new hormone levels, it
can move between what is known as estrogen dominance and estrogen deficiency. Estrogen dominance occurs when progesterone
levels drop, upsetting the counterbalance between estrogen and
progesterone. Estrogen dominance can cause breast tenderness
and fibroid tumors in the breasts and uterus. Women may gain
weight and experience water retention and excessive menstrual
bleeding. Estrogen deficiency causes some of the more classic
menopausal symptoms—such as hot flashes and night sweats.
Depression and anxiety are often by-products of estrogen deficiency. Many women report mental fuzziness and headaches.[3]

Some women seem to breeze through perimenopause, report-
ing few of the above symptoms of either estrogen dominance or
estrogen deficiency. Others, like myself, can check off many of the
items on both lists. Research points to a correlation between the

experiences of PMS, postpartum depression, and depression during perimenopause. Factors such as sensitivity to hormone levels, a family history of depression, and experiences of chronic stress or abuse during childhood play into this correlation.[4]

Induced Menopause

Induced, or artificial, menopause happens when women undergo chemotherapy or radiation in their pelvic area or when the ovaries are removed. When this happens, the body does not have time to adjust. Women are abruptly thrown into menopause. It is estimated that one out of every four American women will experience induced menopause.[5]

The shock of dramatic hormonal changes makes the symptoms of induced menopause extreme, to the point of debilitation. Women experiencing induced menopause need the support of a competent physician and closely monitored hormone replacement therapy.

Premature Menopause

When menopause begins before the age of forty, it is referred to as premature menopause. Premature menopause is caused by early ovarian failure, which may be the result of chronic illnesses, nutritional deficiency, or high levels of stress. The duration of premature menopause is usually shorter than that of natural menopause, lasting from one to three years. The symptoms of premature menopause include mood swings, vaginal dryness, cognitive changes, hot flashes, decreased sexual drive, and sleep disturbances.[6] Currently, there is no treatment to reverse or prevent premature menopause. Because the changes happen so rapidly, women experiencing premature menopause need good medical care along with the support of hormone replacement therapy.

Menopause: A History of Fear

Perhaps you are as I once was—both vaguely aware and fearful of menopause. You may know women who ventured into menopause only to fall apart. You watched in horror as their perfectly orchestrated lives unraveled amid anger, tears, and rage. *You fear you may be one of these women.*

Or you may know women who seemed to breeze through menopause. They deny ever having hot flashes, night sweats, and intense mood swings. *You fear you will not be one of these women.*

As women look ahead toward the land of menopause, we experience a vague sense of foreboding doom. Something tells us it is not going to be pretty. Deep down in our corporate psyche is an encoded message: Be afraid. Be very afraid. This message was left there from the trauma of our foremothers, many of whom endured unbelievable prejudice.

Throughout the centuries, women have endured a great deal of superstition surrounding their bodies in general and menopause in particular. In 1710, the physician Simon David Titius defined menopause as "the worst of all the calamities to beset a sex that seems destined to support the largest share of human misery."[7]

In 1857, the renowned physician Edward Tilt published one of the first medical books devoted entirely to menopause. Tilt was the first person to define menopause as *Climacteric*, or "Change of Life." He defined this period of time as the transformation occurring from "irregularities which precede the last menstrual flow, and [ending] with the re-settlement of health."[8] For Tilt, *Climacteric* conveyed what was going on within women—crisis and resettling of life—better than did the word *menopause*.

Tilt believed menopause was a time of suffering and pathology. The uterus, according to Tilt, was "the keystone of mental pathology." He compiled a list of 120 infirmities common to women during the change. Excitement in women was to be avoided at all costs. Tilt made it his aim to keep women calm, even if doing so meant drugging them into a stupor. Sexual urges in menopausal women were signs of what Tilt described as "anomalous if not morbid impulse, depending on either neuralgic or inflammatory affections of the genital organs." Some women, he noted, were "driven to the verge of insanity by ovario-uterine excitement."[9]

During the Victorian era (1837–1901), the word *hysteria* became the catchall for many menopausal infirmities, including but not limited to depression, bloating, ill temper, and a "tendency to cause trouble."[10] One physician, writing in 1859, claimed that a quarter of all women suffered from hysteria.[11] Another physician developed a catalog of seventy-five pages listing symptoms of hysteria. He pointed out that his list was incomplete![12]

The saga of "women's hysteria" is a sad tale, culminating in the early twentieth-century practice of placing women diagnosed with the malady in mental asylums. Here they were forced into submitting to treatments such as electric shock and ice baths. Because the ovaries were considered the source of hysteria, women underwent unnecessary and dangerous surgery to remove their ovaries. By 1906, more than 150,000 women had undergone an ovariotomy.[13]

In 1895, Alexander Skene, in *Medical Gynecology: A Treatise on the Diseases of Women from the Standpoint of the Physician*, described menopause as "the death of the woman in the woman."[14] This phrase became popular not only among physicians but also among the general population. It aptly put into words everyone's opinion of postmenopausal women. They were the walking dead.

During the early twentieth century, menopause was further medicalized. Research concerning the human endocrine system gave physicians new ways of treating women with menopausal symptoms. Estrogen, in particular, became the hormone that most aptly defined femininity. With the development of synthetic estrogen, it became possible for women to maintain high levels of this hormone through what became known as hormone replacement therapy (HRT). HRT (now referred to as hormone therapy or HT) became the magic pill that cured "the disease" of menopause.

In spite of advancements in science and research, deep-rooted prejudices against older women remained. Medicine provided new weapons of discrimination. At an address to the American College of Surgeons in 1964, gynecologist Robert Kistner used shock effect to gain attention by saying, "We are keeping women around too long—they should all be dead soon after age 45." He went on to explain: "Women are the only mammalian females to live beyond their reproductive usefulness. So it is, by that evolutionary standard that they live too long. But since we do keep them around, we should recognize that during menopause they are living in a state of hormonal imbalance, and we should treat it. We should give them 'the pills' to control the uncomfortable symptoms that women have complained about for centuries."[15]

In 1966, Robert Wilson, a Manhattan gynecologist, published *Feminine Forever*. His book became wildly popular and helped set the stage for the belief that HRT could help women remain "fully feminine—physically and emotionally—for as long as they live."[16] "At age 50," wrote Wilson in 1963 for the *Journal of the American Geriatric Society*, "there are no ova, no follicles, no theca, no estrogen—truly a galloping catastrophe." But with continued estrogen, "breasts and genital organs will not shrivel. Such women will be much more pleasant to live with and will not become dull and unattractive."[17]

During most of the latter part of the twentieth century, a great deal of shame continued to surround the topic of menopause. Menopause was viewed as a medical condition, and women quietly discussed their symptoms with their physicians, most of whom were male. Many women were given large doses of hormone therapy only to learn later of the potential dangers of high levels of estrogen. These dangers include higher risk of heart attack, stroke, and other serious health problems.[18]

The Good News: Times Are Changing

It wasn't too long ago that menopausal women lived in shame and fear. Even now, in some segments of society, a stigma is still attached to the topic of menopause. But there is good news! Since the early 1990s, remarkable strides have been made in research on menopause and women's midlife transition. This research is available to us in very accessible forms and holds promise for our menopausal journeys to be very different from the ones experienced by our foremothers.

In particular, two developments have helped advance both the understanding and the treatment of menopause: the development of bioidentical hormone replacement therapy and a more holistic view of menopause as a time of transformation.

Bioidentical Hormone Replacement Therapy

At the dawn of the twenty-first century, bioidentical hormone replacement therapy came at the right time for many women caught in the dilemma of making a decision regarding HT. Bioidentical hormones are synthesized in labs but are made from hormone precursors found in soybeans or yams. Their molecular structure is more closely identical to the hormones found in the human body. Studies have shown that women experience fewer side effects with bioidentical hormone replacement therapy than with traditional therapies.

In recent years, women have become more involved in decisions regarding HT. They research the differences between traditional HT, such as Premarin, and bioidentical HT. They seek out physicians willing to work in tandem with them to find the best, customized approach to HT. They make decisions as to the strength of their HT regime. Some choose a dusting of hormones, while others go for a more robust treatment. And they make decisions regarding the length of their HT. Some opt for a temporary fix, while others choose the long haul.

Menopause as Transformation

In 1991, Gail Sheehy published her groundbreaking book *Menopause: The Silent Passage*.[19] While integrating the medical aspects of menopause, the book opened the door to discussions of menopause as a time of transformation and explored how menopause can be "a gateway to the second half of life." The book hit a nerve with aging baby boomers looking for ways to continue a rich and full life beyond menopause. "As the pacesetters among baby boom generation women discover menopause on their horizon, they are bringing it out of the closet."[20]

Sheehy offered the idea that women can "become masters of their own menopause," freeing themselves of a one-size-fits-all approach to this time of life.[21] Women no longer needed to blindly follow the prescriptive advice of male physicians. Instead, they could educate themselves regarding the transformation going on within their bodies and the treatments available for menopausal symptoms. They could custom design their menopausal journey.

Ten years after the publication of Sheehy's book, Christiane Northrup, a medical doctor specializing in women's health, helped to advance the understanding of menopause as a time of transformation. Her book *The Wisdom of Menopause*[22] quickly became a *New York Times* bestseller. Northrup's research continues to help women approach menopause as a transition involving physical, social, emotional, and spiritual aspects of life. Today, *The Wisdom of Menopause* is the bible for information on menopause.

While Sheehy wanted to help women master their menopause, Northrup desires to help women work in tandem with menopausal transformation. In her estimation, menopause is a natural process, and the more we learn its secrets and rhythms, the better off our journey through menopause will be.

Thanks to researchers such as Sheehy and Northrup, people are beginning to understand that menopause is not "the death of the woman in the woman." Medical professionals and psychologists are gaining a better understanding of menopause as a time of transformation, "the birth of the woman in the woman." What was once a dead-end street is now being seen as the doorway into the second half of life, a period that can be filled with energy, wisdom, and personal power.

Like Sheehy and Northrup, I write with the assumption that menopause is a time of remarkable transformation. I believe the change offers what James Loder describes as a "transforming moment."[23] Transforming moments are those experiences that radically alter our perceptions of reality. As we encounter transforming moments, we are changed from one way of existing to another. Life is a journey of transforming moments—a time in which things break apart—followed by repatterning and putting things back together.

Menopause is much more than a time of biological change. It is more than a time for focusing on hormones and our physical bodies. It is a crisis containing multiple dimensions, including the psychological and the spiritual. Menopause is a time of life that is ripe with Holy Spirit moments—events initiated and maintained by God's transforming grace. The goal of the menopausal journey is not that we merely adapt but that we are transformed into a new way of being in the world. These moments can be frightening. We are prone to say, "Better to live in the world we know than the one we don't know." It is normal to be afraid of the crisis that is menopause. But know that resisting transformation leads to stagnation. Moreover, we are not alone in this journey. Writes Loder, "The appearance of the Holy One in Scripture is repeatedly accompanied by words of assurance, 'Be not afraid.' The Holy intends to renew and restore."[24]

Developmental Tasks of Menopause

Menopause is a time not only of multidimensional transformation but also of significant developmental tasks. Developmental tasks are simply the accommodations we need to make in order to facilitate further growth. At certain points in life, our psyches begin signaling that things need to change, and either we accommodate to make way for the new and to grow or we resist change and stagnate. Each stage of life has its own set of developmental tasks. For instance, babies face the developmental tasks of learning to crawl, walk, and talk. Adolescents face the tasks of individuating from family and finding their identity. Young adulthood is a time for establishing intimacy, independence, and a career.

Menopause offers its own unique set of developmental tasks. Sue Monk Kidd describes midlife as a time of "developmental transitions." These transitions "are like the tapered neck of an hour glass—difficult but necessary passages that we have to navigate in order to emerge into the next era of life."[25]

I offer *Seven Transforming Gifts of Menopause* as a guide for claiming the opportunities for transformation during menopause.

In this transforming season, you will face seven developmental tasks:

+ Uncovering the repressed and hidden parts of your life
+ Getting in touch with your anger
+ Recovering your authentic self
+ Living in expanded time
+ Claiming your spiritual freedom
+ Embracing a holy vision (calling)
+ Returning to your courageous dragon self

I refer to these developmental tasks as gifts because each task, once accomplished, moves you closer to becoming more mature, courageous, and wise.

Each gift (developmental task) opens the door for others to follow. For instance, the gift of uncovering sets the stage for you to claim the gift of anger. The gift of anger makes it easier to identify your authentic self. The gift of the authentic self makes it easier to move into a world of expanded time. The gift of expanded time opens the way for the gift of spiritual freedom. After finding the gift of spiritual freedom, you will be ready to embrace a holy vision—calling—for the second half of life. All these gifts make way for you to enter the dragon's den, where you can find your dragon self and claim your gift of courage.

You may be one of those lucky women who breeze through menopause without some of the more distressing symptoms. It is still important for you to achieve menopause's developmental tasks. Successful achievement of these tasks means you will be more fully able to face the challenges of the second half of life.

One of the strengths of human development is its fluidity. If we miss critical developmental windows or fully achieving some of life's developmental tasks, we can always return to those is-sues. If you are a woman past the age of menopause, there is still time to revisit the opportunities hidden in this phase of life. Being past menopause will make achieving the tasks more dif-ficult because your body was primed for transformation during menopause. But don't despair; you can still take advantage of the gifts of menopause!

ONE

PUBERTY AND THE RELATIONAL SELF

PEOPLE WHO LIVE ON THE SEASHORE know that things never stay the same. Tides ebb and flow, ever so slowly altering the coastal landscape. From time to time, furious storms arrive, bringing with them the power to dramatically change the shoreline. The waves and winds of one storm bring in huge amounts of sand, covering houses and filling streets. Other storms wash away the shore, uncovering objects hidden years before.

Like the sea, life is composed of rhythmic ebbs and flows. Ever so slowly, day by day, week by week, month by month, we grow and change. We hardly notice these changes. After several years, we wonder, *Where did the time go? I don't remember aging.*

Then there are other experiences. We sometimes call them crises. These experiences have the power to disrupt and dramatically change everything. Crises are the stormy times in life: a divorce, the death of a beloved family member, the loss of a job, health issues. They stretch our ability to endure, and they demand we make radical adjustments. After a crisis, we can never go back to the way things were.

No one likes crises, but they are often necessary for growth. We are transformed through crisis. In fact, disruption is built into our DNA. These "embodied crises" arrive on cue, disrupting our normal way of being in the world. When a baby experiences teething, the very area of her body that gives so much pleasure, the mouth, turns against her. In response, she cries and seeks someone to take away the pain. But the pain signals that teeth are breaking through the gums. These teeth will open an avenue to reach a new milestone—eating solid food!

Puberty is one of those DNA-coded crises. On the outskirts of puberty, deep in the recesses of the brain, hormonal shifts begin to occur. The young girl hardly notices these changes at first, but before long her body is awash with hormonal changes. She notices. Everyone notices. Prior to puberty, she was a child. After puberty, she is a young woman. Before puberty, she did not have menstrual periods. Now the young woman has a period every month. Before puberty, her chest was flat. After puberty, she has enlarged breasts.

What we do not often see is how puberty changes a young woman's psyche. Before puberty, she thought and acted one way. After puberty, her sense of self and the way she relates to people are dramatically changed. The brain/hormonal changes of puberty have altered the young woman's entire being. As much as a young woman might want to, she can never return to childhood.

After puberty, things settle down for a long while, and the young woman eventually turns into a middle-aged woman. She comes to believe she will always be the kind of person she has been since puberty. She has settled nicely into the rhythmic swell of the tides of her menstrual cycle. She slowly ages. It seems life will continue on as usual. But just as she was unaware of the early changes signaling the storm of puberty, she may be unaware that deep down in the recesses of her brain the storm of perimenopause is brewing. After a while, these changes become more dramatic, and she is forced to take notice of the transformation her body is undergoing.

Just as the storm of puberty transformed the girl into a young woman, the storm of perimenopause transforms the middle-aged woman into a mature woman. This mature woman will think differently than her younger self. The younger woman could easily brush aside things, letting them go for the sake of relational harmony. The mature woman takes notice of things. The younger woman was keenly attuned to the voices of others, to the point of ignoring her own truth. The mature woman begins to listen to her own voice. After a while, the menopausal woman is no longer the woman she once was—physically, mentally, or emotionally.

The dramatic transformation women undergo during perimenopause and menopause is the focus of this book. However, before you can understand what is happening to you during this time of your life, you need to take a look back at your younger self. For that reason, this chapter is included to help you understand the powerful crisis of puberty. Although you are long past this upheaval, it is important to know what happens to girls during this time so that you will be able to interpret how the changes shaped you into the woman you are today.

The Perfect Storm of Puberty

The crisis that arrives at puberty blows the door open to adulthood. I call it a perfect storm because two frontal systems—societal pressures and biological changes—converge into one gigantic maelstrom. The perfect storm of puberty arrives bearing the gift of the relational self. The relational self views the world from within a web of relationships woven together with tight cords of responsibility. The relational self is that part of a woman willing to forgo her own interests for the interests and needs of others.

The self of a young girl, the one you often see during childhood, is the "I." She pretty much sees herself as the lead actor in the world. She may be talkative, assertive, and overly confident. She has friends, enjoys school, and wants to run for president of the United States.

The relational self created at puberty submerges the "I" in order to become the "not I" or the "we." This young woman is often less talkative and less assertive and sees herself as the supporting actor. She may have forgotten about running for president.

JANA

When Jana was ten, she was fearless, winsome, self-assured, and a bit mischievous. Every time she entered a room it seemed that she owned the space. Jana was an engaging conversationalist who had an opinion about everything. I loved being around her, partly because she reminded me of my own ten-year-old self.

Jana's parents lived in another state, so I wasn't with her very often. In fact, I did not see Jana at all between the ages of ten and thirteen. After Jana had turned thirteen, her parents invited me to their home for dinner. On the drive to their house, I braced myself for their daughter's larger-than-life personality. Upon entering my friends' home, I spotted Jana immediately. She was busily setting the table for dinner.

As Jana set the table, we talked. I soon realized that this young woman was not the child I remembered. In the outspoken girl's place was a very pleasant and somewhat hesitant young woman. I never would have used the words *nice* or *sweet* to describe ten-year-old Jana, but these words aptly described the person in the dining room that evening.

During our conversation, what struck me most was the change in Jana's voice. The voice of ten-year-old Jana had a deep quality that made every sentence declarative. This young woman's voice was softly modulated. Her voice lilted upward at the end of her sentences, as if to say, "Don't take anything I say very seriously." Most unnerving was the high-pitched nervous laugh that filled the silence between Jana's sentences. After a while, I became anxious to end our conversation. It had become so painful that I wanted to shake her and scream, "Where did you go?!"

At dinner that evening, I mentioned how much I missed Jana's outspoken demeanor. Her father spoke up quickly. "That girl was a handful, wasn't she? I thought she would never grow up." I prayed no one at the table heard the deep sigh that escaped from me.

The Storm Front of Societal Pressure

Although I was startled at the transformation that had taken place in Jana between the ages of ten and thirteen, I should have expected to see a different girl than the one I remembered. Jana was undergoing the perfect storm of puberty. Two storm fronts, societal pressure and biological changes, had converged on this unsuspecting young woman.

The front of societal pressure was bearing down hard on Jana. She was surrounded by images of womanhood telling her she must become less assertive and less direct: "Be a nice girl and behave yourself." As a child, Jana did not notice the pressures to act more mature. She chose to ignore the caution to "lower her voice" or "be more like a girl." She was too busy being herself to cave in to the pressure. Somehow, somewhere between the ages of ten and thirteen, she began to get the message: If I want to be accepted and liked, I must become a nice girl.

Jana's family is part of a culture that believes women were created to be submissive and loving caregivers of men and families. By

21

the time Jana turned thirteen, she had listened to many sermons about "a woman's place" in the home and in the church. While Jana's family and church systems were willing to put up with a young girl's energy, voice, and drive, they would not tolerate this type of young woman. At a certain point, Jana was expected to "grow up" and put her childish ways behind her.

Jana attended a large middle school in the suburbs of a southern city. This environment reinforced the idea that popularity, especially with boys, meant developing "a feminine personality." The outspoken girl of elementary school was not welcome in a middle school world where girls are valued for their beauty and body size, not their voice.

Jana's experiences during her transition into puberty are not unusual. At this time, peers, the media, and societal images begin to have more influence than they did during childhood. In addition, when young girls arrive at adolescence, they are handed a powerful script narrating a story of what it means to be feminine. This narrative is everywhere—media, schools, communities of faith, and family systems. Girls cannot escape it.

Mary Pipher, a noted psychologist and researcher of girls' development, points out that during adolescence, girls are given the terrible choice of being either feminine or adult. They cannot be both. Writes Pipher, "Now girls are expected to sacrifice the parts of themselves that our culture considers masculine on the altar of social acceptability and to shrink their souls down to a petite size."[1]

Attributes such as risk taking, assertiveness, and self-confidence are not welcome in a world where women are expected to be compliant, nice, and supporting of others. Girls like Jana, who have strong inclinations toward what is often described as a more masculine side, have a hard time adjusting to expectations that they leave these parts of their identity back in the world of childhood.

Bruno Bettelheim analyzed the "young women's disappearance scenario"—a common occurrence in classic fairy tales.[2] In these stories, upon entering puberty, young men leave home for the hero's quest. On this quest, they conquer dragons and engage in conflict with other males, all the while discovering their place in the world. But at the onset of puberty, young women—such as Sleeping Beauty and Snow White—are cursed to fall asleep. While in this deep slumber, they lie in wait for the arrival of a prince whose kiss provides intimacy. In finding intimacy, the young woman discovers her identity.

Fairy tales reveal how images of young women as passive sleepers are deeply embedded in the human psyche. These stories narrate expectations that girls do not go on a quest for identity. Instead, at puberty, girls enter into a limbo phase, a time of living life in neutral and waiting for the arrival of a young man. Love and marriage bring the gift of intimacy and, as a by-product, identity.

Adolescent girls are given the choice of being authentic, with the possibility of being scorned, or feminine, with the possibility of being loved. Part of being feminine is locking their questing, adventurous selves in the deep chambers of their psyches. In their places emerges the pleasing young woman, a seeming self. The seeming self becomes adept at anticipating the expectations of others and matching those expectations. "At adolescence, girls go down in droves," laments Pipher, "crashing and burning in a social and developmental Bermuda Triangle."[3]

JENNIFER

Jennifer, a student in one of my classes, spoke so softly that I had to lean forward to hear her. After a few weeks of being put off by the softness of her voice, I encouraged her to speak louder. In response, Jennifer told me her sad story. As a young girl, she had what she called "a loud mouth." When she was thirteen, Jennifer's male Sunday school teacher told her that God did not approve of girls who spoke loudly. He warned, "God will give you throat cancer if you do not learn to speak more softly, like a woman." His words hit their intended target. Out of fear, Jennifer's voice went underground.

I could tell Jennifer was an intelligent and gifted young woman. Her written work was stellar. But she lacked self-confidence, especially in the classroom and in social settings. Sadly, I could never get her to find her repressed voice. In fact, seminary was too much for her. After one semester, she dropped out.

The Storm Front of Brain/Hormonal Changes

The thirteen-year-old Jana I encountered was a young woman undergoing transformation that was partly due to cultural pressure to conform to images of femininity. However, not everything happening to her was related to outside forces. Jana was also experiencing remarkable biological changes. The abusive remarks of Jennifer's Sunday school teacher came at the right time in her life to hit their mark, when she was also experiencing remarkable biological changes. Had he made them when she was nine, she may have had the ego strength to ignore him.

Women have long been victimized by opinions regarding their biological nature. As discussed in the introduction, history is littered with superstitious beliefs about women's biological destiny. No one wants to go back there! By the last quarter of the twentieth century, due to strides in science and advancements in understanding gender, the idea that biology is destiny had gone out of favor. For the first time in history, women were not deemed to be biologically deficit or "misbegotten males." We could all take a deep breath and talk about what it means to be human.

During this time period, discussions regarding gender differences were muted because of the fear that "difference" could be used to prove male superiority. We can be grateful for this era. It gave us space to focus on societal factors contributing to women's development. It allowed us to critically analyze how women were shaped by cultural images of the feminine.

In recent years, while continuing to focus on what it means to be human, researchers of gender have dared to venture back into discussions regarding women's differences. Unlike those of previous generations, these researchers approach their study with the idea that different does not mean inferior. Neither do they follow the Freudian dictum that biology is destiny. Instead, they try to weave together sociological and biological dynamics into a more holistic vision of women's identity.

In 1982, Carol Gilligan's book *In a Different Voice* became a game changer in discussions of gender differences.[4] Her research challenged old assumptions that women's valuing of relationships and care was inferior to masculine images of independence and achievement. Gilligan's groundbreaking work gave permission for women to own the ethics of care and to claim their valuing of interdependence. It was okay for women to say "we" and to see themselves in a connected web of life.

Christiane Northrup is a researcher who has brought biology back to the front burner in regard to discussions of women's development. "The process of sublimating our truest selves begins early in adolescence," writes Northrup. "A young woman's 'activist' mindset, her forthrightness, and honesty all become hormonally sublimated."[5] Northrup advocates acknowledging these factors while paying careful attention to the ways society exploits them.

I believe it is safe to say that while societal pressure is strong enough to alter the identities of adolescent girls, such pressure cannot explain all the dramatic changes that occur in their lives. Girls are swamped with a convergence of expectations from society as well as brain/hormonal changes.

During puberty, the reproductive hormones that stimulate the opioid centers in the female brain become active. They produce what Northrup calls narcotic-like chemicals that provide "a feel-good sensation, a natural high" for women as they bear children and nurture families.[6] This feel-good sensation is fueled as estrogen rises during the high fertility phase of the menstrual cycle. In addition, the hormones prolactin and oxytocin flood a woman's system during her mothering mode of breast-feeding and nurturing children. This flood of hormones provides a sense of contentment and fulfillment that continues throughout the childbearing years.

The hormonal shifts in adolescence are powerful forces stimulating a desire for sex, intimacy, and children. They create a sense of well-being in women, a reward system of sorts, for the processes of sexual relations and childbearing. They help create what is known as the nesting syndrome. In the warm flood of brain chemistry, young women are drawn into a world where they find great fulfillment in marriage, family, and homemaking.

These brain changes, combined with cultural rewards, help women desire and maintain the life of marriage and children. They work to facilitate women who work for stability in relationships. They make it easier for them to overlook injustice for the sake of relational harmony. These changes also make it easier for women to conform to societal forces that feed them images of the good wife and the caring mother.

Honoring the Relational Self

I met my husband, Jackie, in a philosophy class during college. We began our journey together discussing and arguing about the various branches of this academic discipline. Shortly after the birth of our first daughter, Jackie began a discussion on educational philosophy. I recall sitting there and nursing our beautiful newborn baby, looking at him, and wondering how he could be so interested in philosophy at a time like this. This time of my life was filled with the joys, travails, and challenges of motherhood and the wonder and pain of nursing. In light of these events, educational philosophy seemed boring and speculative.

I went on to get a PhD and to become a tenured professor. Clearly, my lack of interest in philosophy didn't last. I must admit there were times in my quest for advanced education when I had to push not only against societal expectations of the good mother but also against my own body. Sometimes I felt like two different people: the nurturing wife and mother and the academic professor.

The hormonal covering over or sublimating of the self that occurs in puberty is a gift. It is a gift to families, communities, and societies that women desire to be in intimate relationships with others. Without the desire for relationships, we may never become nurturing wives and mothers! For that reason, we should be kind to that part of us that once made us willing to totally immerse ourselves in child-rearing and in creating a home. Moreover, we need to be kind to women who find fulfillment in these roles.

As much as we should honor the abilities of women to generate care, let's be careful not to stereotype women into relational images. There are many women who do not have strong nurturing urges. There are women who, like myself, choose to have both a career and children. During the short time spans when I was not teaching, I became depressed. Staying at home full time was toxic for me. I found fulfillment by combining teaching and mothering. Some women never marry. Some women find the idea of being a nurturer or a caregiver as contrary to their authentic self. All choices should be honored.

Furthermore, the knowledge that hormonal shifts help to sublimate young women's drive for independence is not an excuse to keep these women hidden away or to refuse them the power of self-direction. In fact, it is during this time that adolescent girls need extra encouragement to develop a strong core identity. The push and pull of society combined with hormonal changes in the body make this difficult for them to do alone.

Parents should honor their daughter's interpersonal concerns. The ethics of care and inclusion should be cultivated in young women. At the same time, it is especially important to help girls claim their identity apart from relationships. Parents, the right schools, and communities of faith can make the critical difference between a girl getting forever lost in the Bermuda Triangle of early adolescence and a girl navigating through the storm and emerging on the other side with an intact sense of self. It is hard, but not impossible, for girls to become a unique gestalt of the "I" and the "not I" (we).

I agree with Jean Baker Miller's hunch regarding women's interpersonal identity. She argues that women's relational sense of self "contains the possibilities for an entirely different (and more advanced) approach to living and functioning . . . [in which] affiliation is valued as highly as, or more highly than, self-enhancement."[7] Relational identity creates healthy people; it creates healthy communities. In order for women to contribute to an advanced way of human community, we have to make sure that this interpersonal identity is solidly grounded in a secure and confident ego identity.

Otherwise, women will continue to serve primarily as support-givers in the human drama.

A Time for Grace

My adolescence occurred during the turbulent 1960s. I am grateful that by this time the second wave of feminism provided young women an alternative script to the more traditional narrative. The feminist script encouraged young women to enter the public sphere and help change the world. Commercials on television told us we could be all we wanted to be. Many of my generation heeded this call. Large numbers of us went to college and chose careers outside of traditional "feminine" careers.

Despite the feminist movement, the traditional female script was still very powerful, especially in certain conservative segments of society. As a consequence, many women of my generation heard two starkly different messages: the message of society to be all we wanted to be and the message of church and local communities to be the silent "help meet" God had designed women to be. Some women, like myself, embraced the feminist script. We did not see it as contrary to our faith or to our nature as women. Other women rejected the feminist narrative, believing it to be an attempt to destroy the foundations of family life.

In the midst of all the tension between traditional and feminist ideas, women of my era learned to coexist. We raised families and managed our lives. At times, conflicting scripts about what makes "a real woman" created dissonance within us, pulling us in two different directions. At other times, these scripts caused battles among us. Many women of my generation were caught in the drama of the mommy wars—working mothers versus stay-at-home mothers. And, yes, each side was often unkind to the other.

I remember being strident in my criticisms of women who gave up college to settle into their roles as full-time homemakers and mothers. I also have painful memories of facing the passive-aggressive criticisms of other women: "You must know your children really miss their mother when you travel [a long pause for emphasis], I hope they don't suffer too much damage."

As we enter menopause, much of the unfinished business of our earlier lives returns to haunt us. Standing at the threshold of the second half of life, we bring all this baggage with us. It is time to make peace with our past and with one another.

A while back, I had a conversation with a woman about the choices we made as young women. She had taken the traditional route of stay-at-home mother. I had taken the path of both mother and career woman. I confessed to this woman how bad I felt when other women criticized me for working outside the home. "I would have been one of those women," she admitted. She went on to explain that, while she believed her chosen path was right for her, she regretted criticizing others for taking a different one. Likewise, I confessed I would have criticized her for not having a career outside her family. Now I honored her choice. At that moment, the two of us found a measure of grace.

As you enter menopause, pause to reflect on the decisions you made as a young woman. Try to remember what it was like to be twenty-five and full of life, love, and energy. What idealistic images did you have of marriage, family, and career? On the down side, perhaps you also navigated the mommy wars. What wounds did you receive during those wars? What scars do you still carry? Who did you wound?

Maybe you decided not to marry or not to have children. At the time you were making the decision, you chose with awareness of what was best for you. Perhaps you always wanted a husband and

30

children but never had the opportunity. Whatever decisions you made, whatever decisions were made for you, now is the time to give yourself grace. Now is the time to give grace to others. There is another storm on the horizon, and in order to face it, you will need to lighten the load and trim your sails.

Personal Reflection Activities

1. Take time to remember what it was like to navigate the storm of puberty. Describe the intensity of your emotions. What was it like to want desperately to fit in? Do you recall the pressures to conform to images of a nice girl? Describe this girl. Perhaps you can recall what was expected of you to be considered feminine. What did feminine look like to you then?

2. If you grew up in a conservative culture, you may have faced the added pressure to accept your "place" as a woman. You may have been told that you were designed by God to be a certain way and to fulfill certain roles. This "certain way" may have been counter to the person you were as an older child. If so, what parts of your self did you have to let go of in order to become acceptable? What parts of your self went missing when you began to conform?

3. Consider your voice. How would you describe it? Do you speak with an upward lilt? In what ways are your sentences structured so as not to be threatening? Do you have a nervous laugh that surfaces in the silence between sentences? Why do you think you developed this silence filler?

4. What decisions did you make as a young woman that you now regret? Do you tend to be harsh toward your younger self? Why? Try to remember what it felt like to be that young woman and offer grace regarding her decisions.

5. What words describe the image of God that you had when you were a child? Did this image change when you entered adulthood or did it remain the same? If it changed, what words would you now use to describe God?

6. What parts of your self seemed to disappear into a Bermuda Triangle? How might they be seeking to return?

Group Reflection Activities

1. As a group, brainstorm—think aloud—about the words you would use to describe your adolescence. In brainstorming, there are no bad words or good words. There are no correct words or incorrect words. Have someone record these words on a white board or a large piece of paper taped to the wall. Take a minute to reflect on the words. Note the words you have in common with others.

2. Divide into groups of working moms and stay-at-home moms. There could also be groups for those who never married and those who never had children. People should express reasons for why they are in one category or the other. Make no negative comments or judgments regarding the statements made by other women. Take time to really listen to one another. After everyone has shared, take the opportunity to affirm someone on "the other side."

3. Take a few moments to share regrets you may have regarding decisions you made as a young woman. Reflect together on these decisions. Where do you see the threads of grace in one another's lives in spite of the "bad" decisions?

4. End the session by reflecting on the following: How are you the same as you were in childhood? How might menopause be an opportunity to revisit issues from the past?

TWO

THE GIFT
OF UNCOVERING

The shell must be cracked apart if what is in it is to come out, for if you want the kernel, you must break the shell.

—Meister Eckhart, *"Hanc Dicit Dominus"*

Dorothy stood in the doorway with Toto in her arms, and looked at the sky. . . . Suddenly Uncle Henry stood up. "There's a cyclone coming, Em," he called. . . . There came a great shriek from the wind, and the house shook so hard Dorothy lost her footing. . . . The great pressure of the wind on every side of the house raised it up higher and higher, until it was at the very top of the cyclone; and there it remained and was carried miles and miles away.

—Frank L. Baum, *The Wizard of Oz*

AS WE WOMEN AGE, we tend to forget the angst, intensity of emotions, and first stirrings of desire that were part of the perfect storm of puberty. Time passes, things settle down, and we begin to think the life created by this storm will last forever. We bleed, bear children, nurture our families, work every day, all the while not giving much thought to that coded biological clock that continues to tick. Its ticking moves us closer and closer toward another maelstrom.

We don't post a sentry on lookout for the approaching storm. If we did, we might take note of the small swells of changes in our monthly cycle, the unexplained weight gain, or the dark clouds of depression on the horizon. Most often we drift along unaware of the approaching storm of perimenopause. But then it arrives, and its gale-force winds and large waves force us to pay attention.

The storm of perimenopause brings the first gift of menopause—the gift of uncovering. Its winds and waves have the power to uncover aspects of our lives that went missing years before. This storm offers an opportunity to revisit the past and to remake the future. It arrives with relentless force and is intent on laying bare the forgotten, the repressed, and the overlooked. This is the storm that blows open the door to the second half of life.

EVELYN

Evelyn and I are a great deal alike. We both chose careers in higher education, and each of us has assumed leadership roles in the academy. Evelyn is around ten years older than I; she is someone I looked to as a mentor and role model. It was my opinion that Evelyn was the consummate eternal optimist. She had a way of seeing the bright side of everyone and everything. I often wished I could be more like her.

A few years ago, my perception of Evelyn came to a crashing end. I was in New York City for a conference. Having seen Evelyn's name on the program, I was anxious to spend some time with her. Soon after arriving in the ballroom of the conference hotel, I spotted Evelyn standing at a table. I remember anticipating the warmth of her vibrant personality. But as I neared her, Evelyn turned and looked my way. I was startled by the look on her face. It was a look I had never seen on her—a look of absolute rage.

Later that evening, while talking over dinner, Evelyn spilled out a litany of disappointments. She talked about being overlooked for advancement in rank. She talked about being pushed out of an organization she had founded. She poured out anger at her university, church, family, and almost everyone in her life. I was shocked. All I could do was listen, nod my head, and try to affirm her. I wondered what had happened to the optimistic Evelyn I once knew.

Looking back and reflecting on this event, I believe I encountered Evelyn during the rough phase of perimenopause. She was at a point in her life where she could no longer suppress the negative, and her usual spirit of bright optimism gave way to brooding anger.

Facing the Bill Collector

When we are young, most of our energy is focused on what Richard Rohr calls "the first half of life tasks."[1] These developmental tasks include establishing a career, getting married, raising children, and becoming economically stable. In the first half of life, we have little time to focus on things such as remaining true to our authentic selves. We are too busy expending our energy on others.

While living in the first half of life, we might find it easy to let go of things that offend us. We let these things go because we are busy. We let them go to avoid conflict. We let them go because there is not enough emotional energy to deal with them. We fail to realize we never really let go of things; we merely deposit them deep in our psyches.

"Throughout a woman's childbearing years," writes Christiane Northrup, "a kind of 'debt account' is established where existing and future issues accumulate, compounding interest with each passing month that the debt goes unpaid."[2] The storm of perimenopause is the bill collector on this unpaid debt.

The bill collector comes calling by causing dramatic changes in a woman's brain chemistry, altering the delicate interaction between the hypothalamus, the pituitary gland, the ovaries, and the key hormones that are produced in these areas. The body's attempts to navigate this upheaval create a rough ride for most women.

Up to the time of perimenopause, the body's balance of hormones is designed for childbearing. At the approach of perimenopause, progesterone levels drop, thereby upsetting the normal balance of estrogen and progesterone. The body reacts by seeking a new normal. It may take a while for a woman's body to find its new hormonal balance. Until that time, it is not uncommon for a woman to experience symptoms such as breast swelling, heavy menstrual periods, fibroids in the breasts and uterus, frequent urinary tract infections, and vaginal dryness. These are all physical changes that signal a woman has entered perimenopause.

The physical symptoms are only part of this powerful storm. The transformation going on in the brain also disrupts the warm, nurturing feelings that characterize a woman's earlier life. These warm feelings are replaced with other strong forces such as vivid memories, anger, and intensity of thought.

During perimenopause, women pay attention to things they once overlooked or glossed over for the sake of harmony in relationships. This focus of attention happens due to changes in the hormone GnRH (gonadotropin-releasing hormone). At perimenopause, the GnRH, produced in the hypothalamus, primes the brain for new perception. It works in tandem with estrogen and progesterone to bring out stored and repressed memories. Things long forgotten bubble up to the surface.[3]

Perimenopausal women are often characterized as overreacting and emotional. They are not overreacting. They are no longer viewing the world through a cloud of hormones produced during their childbearing years. The brain that once facilitated sublimation of anger for the sake of harmony gives way to one that is ready to deal with life's unfinished business. As a new hormonal balance emerges, women begin to take note of the disparity in power, injustice in society, betrayal in relationships, and disappointments that they once were willing to overlook. In other words, the rose-colored glasses come off.

During perimenopause, a woman's brain is awash with hormonal changes—changes that are as intense as the ones that occurred during puberty. The changes during puberty had the effect of sublimating identity for the sake of harmony. Now the powerful hormonal shifts are working in reverse, pushing the seeming self to give way to make space for the authentic self to return.

During puberty, your authentic self did not disappear. She was merely buried beneath a lovely wash of hormones. Once this level of hormones begins to shift, your self—the one who climbed trees or played soccer, the one who played with dragons, the one who owned the world—is awakened. She is no longer content to be banished to the hidden caverns of your psyche. She is insistent that her return will not go unnoticed. Let's just say she has some unresolved issues.

The waves of biological changes, as they wash over a woman's body, seek to leave no stone unturned. The pain and anger, once so easy to repress, begin to make their presence known. At times, a woman will have no control over the tears that stream down her face. She may be shocked at the intensity of her emotions. She does not have this storm—it has her.

To complicate matters, the storm of perimenopause seems to come at the most inopportune time. It often arrives when women are facing the empty nest and the care of aging parents. Or it might occur when we are trying to deal with the difficulties of raising teenagers who are going through hormonal changes of their own. It is for these very reasons that we are given the wake-up call. Our bodies are letting us know that our previous existence cannot contain the world that is coming. We must be born again.

During this rough period, it is tempting to seek hormone therapy (HT) to alleviate the symptoms entirely. Such a desire is easily understood. We want to return to a life characterized by a measure of control. We want our bodies to return to normal. We want to love everyone again. We want to be happy again. We want to return to the security of the relational matrix.

Some of my friends have told me stories about pleading with their physicians for drugs during perimenopause. They just wanted something to make it all go away. I know one woman who asked her physician for the highest dose of HT available. When told of the possible side effects, she agreed to sign papers stating that she would not hold her physician responsible for any serious effects of the drugs. "I just want my life back," she told me.

The problem that needs to be addressed is not our hormone levels. It is our anger levels. HT has a place in curbing some of the more severe symptoms of hot flashes, anxiety attacks, and depression. Sometimes the symptoms of perimenopause are so dramatic that maintaining regular routines of life without help from HT is difficult. But Northrup cautions women not to overmedicate. She notes that medicating the anger to maintain the status quo is killing the messenger.[4]

My own perimenopause was so rough that I worked with my physician to find the right dose of natural hormone therapy. After doing blood work, he prescribed for me a combination of estrogen, progesterone, and a tiny bit of androgen testosterone. Taking this combination allowed me to overcome some of the severe symptoms of night sweats and anxiety attacks. But my dose of HT did not radically alter my body's hormonal chemistry, returning it to the levels of premenopause. In other words, I did not get to bypass the storm.

HT can provide a more stable backdrop to perimenopause, but it should not replace the life cleaning that needs to be done for us to move into a healthier and more fulfilling life. Life cleaning is difficult. No one wants to open the doors to musty and dark places where memories are stored. But if we allow the winds and the waves of this storm to do their cleansing work, our lives will be transformed. We will be ready to face the doorway leading to the second half of life.

A Word of Caution

When a young girl enters puberty, she faces societal forces that work in tandem with her hormonal changes. Parents don't run to a physician and beg for drugs that will make puberty go away. Instead, they try to help their daughter weather the storm. The pubescent girl is given images (some good and some bad) telling her how important it is for her to become a young woman.

Women experience perimenopause differently. The same cultural influences that encourage young girls to let go of their own identity during puberty are still at work discouraging older women from having separateness, voice, and power. In other words, they want you to remain the young woman created in puberty.

There is little space for the woman being born during the storm of perimenopause. Images of the good wife or the nice girl continue to help maintain the status quo. Angry perimenopausal women are not welcome in such a world. Writes Northrup, "As a woman makes the transition to the second half of her life, she

finds herself in a struggle not only with her own aversion to conflict and confrontation but also with the culture's view of how
women 'should' be."[5]

For these reasons, when we face this storm, we often feel totally
alone. Few support systems are available to help us navigate the
winds of change that are wreaking havoc on our lives. We are
rarely told that perimenopause is another developmental milestone. We are not informed that we are undergoing transformation into a more mature person. Instead, women are encouraged
to view menopause as a medical condition. It is easy for us to
find advice on medication, diet, and exercise, but it is hard to
find advice on preparing for the changes coming in our psyches
and spirits.

To make matters worse, it is hard for us to find safe places
where we can receive emotional and spiritual support during the
storm of perimenopause. Tears are interpreted as a symptom of
weakness and fragility. Spouses find it difficult to support the
questioning, remembering, and anger. Children want their mother
to return to normal. All around us are messages telling us to
get over it or to move on. It is easy to understand why so many
women overmedicate!

Remember this: when not allowed to express anger, the body
turns on itself. "Feelings buried alive do not die; they fester,"
notes Iyania Vanzanti, host of a talk show on OWN network. I
have known women who developed an array of illnesses during
midlife. Sometimes these ailments took over their lives to the
extent that the ailments became their identity. Talking with these
women means listening to a catalog of symptoms, medical tests,
and physicians.

Sadly, it is more acceptable for women to be ill than angry.
There are plenty of derogatory names for women who dare to
express their anger and regret and who point out injustice in

their own lives and in the lives of others. Faced with the possibility of encountering disapproval and name-calling, many women choose to turn their anger inward, swallowing it down in huge, toxic doses. I have more to say about anger in the next chapter.

Women accustomed to hiding their pain and smiling despite their angst are tempted to continue to do so during the storm of perimenopause. This behavior is their default mode. Such women have perfected the art of pleasing others to the degree that it seems to come naturally. They have developed the art of "seeming" to the degree that they no longer know the difference between seeming and being. They fool themselves into believing that their own orchestrated pleasing behavior is the real self. Pleasing, seeming women are willing to work extra hard to repress their pain, often to the point of physical exhaustion.

You may be a woman who long ago gave up being for seeming. You may be a woman who did whatever it took to keep relational harmony. If so, be aware that you will have strong urges to resist the storm of perimenopause, especially its power to uncover things from the past.

Take comfort knowing that this storm is not designed to destroy you. It is designed to destroy your earlier way of being in this world, a space too small for the new life waiting to be born. Sue Monk Kidd makes a striking observation about the book *The Wizard of Oz*. She notes that when the cyclone came, Dorothy was standing on the threshold of a too-small house. "In that moment, she received her call to go on the quest. It came through a crisis swooping down unexpectedly upon her. It was her moment of separation, her moment of opportunity."[6]

While in the storm of perimenopause, it is normal to be conflicted. As you look out over the waves of this terrible storm, you will hear a voice calling you out into the waters. Deep down you know there is something more out there—a richer and more adventurous life. But there is the strong temptation to batten down the hatches and seek safe harbor where you can ride out the storm.

Speaking out of experience with her own midlife struggles, Kidd warns, "We have within us a deep longing to grow and become a new creature, but we possess an equally strong compulsion to remain the same—to burrow in our safe, secure places."[7]

In *The Wizard of Oz*, when the cyclone was bearing down on the house, Dorothy's aunt Em threw open the trap door in the floor. As she ran down the steps into the cellar, she called for Dorothy to follow. During this time of your life, voices other than your own will tell you to choose the safe route. Some of the loudest voices will be the voices of other women. These are the women who chose the safe route, and their voices are often the hardest to resist.

As you stand on the threshold of midlife, watching the maelstrom of perimenopause coming for you, choose well. What appears to be a safe place—namely, the dwelling you have known for many years—can turn from being a place of life to being a place of death. Staying means you will become a shell of your former self, lacking both the life essence of your previous existence and the rich gifts of the life waiting to be born. You will become like a pupa trapped in its cocoon, unable to become the beautiful butterfly of its second half of life. Your menopausal self will be stillborn.

How to Claim the Gift of Uncovering

You may agree it is important to receive the gifts borne by the winds of the storm of perimenopause but wonder how to do so. I know from experience how difficult it is to enter into the mysterious realm of this great unknown. During my own menopausal journey, there were times when I did not know if the person I was becoming would in any way resemble the person I once was. I was often tempted to resist change, hunker down, and endure the storm. After all, I knew how to live in the house of my earlier life. I had no idea how to live if it was demolished.

I am glad I resisted the urges to merely endure the storm of perimenopause. Today, I am in a much healthier place, a place where the tyranny of pleasing and performing no longer dominates my waking hours. I live in a much more peaceful, larger house.

Looking back from the other side of menopause, I have identified two things you can do to make the most of this developmental window: (1) lean into the storm and (2) get in touch with your body.

Lean into the Storm

I often get frustrated observing people "enjoying" the ocean surf. It seems more work than fun. Watching them face the incoming waves, bracing for the big hit, I think about how they are missing the real thrills of the ocean's power. People standing in the crashing surf seem to believe that their bodies can resist the onslaught of the force of water bearing down on them. Sometimes the resistance works, but most times I see a lot of people being knocked down only to stand up again for another round.

As someone who loves to body surf, I prefer the enjoyment that comes in riding the waves instead of resisting them. A huge wave is more powerful than my body. Its force is greater than my resistance. When I jump on top of a wave, just at the moment it is cresting, and ride it to shore, for a few moments I am one with the wave. I am privileged to experience the thrill of its power.

Many women stand in the surf and bravely face the incoming waves of the storm of perimenopause. In doing so, they experience pain beyond what is necessary. This is the pain of being knocked

45

down and swamped by the waves of change that are demanding attention. Christiane Northrup describes the symptoms of perimenopause as "labor pains . . . part of our adaption to the hormonal changes that take place as our biological focus switches from procreation to personal growth."[8] Fighting these pains only makes things worse. In fact, she points out that resistance to the storm of perimenopause can cause the symptoms to last much longer than necessary.

The image of African American women as powerful matriarchs contributes to their sense of well-being and control in their lives. They are the strong ones upon whom others lean during hard times. Here is the paradox: this image can make menopause more difficult. In her book *The Black Woman's Guide to Menopause*, Carolyn Scott Brown writes, "Being powerful and in control can count against us, causing us to make assumptions and jump to premature conclusions."[9]

If you are one of those strong black women, know that it will be incredibly difficult to lean into the storm of perimenopause. Your psyche may have a built-in resistance to giving in. But in order to move into a healthier and more peaceful second half of life, you must let go of the idea that you are invincible. These waves crashing upon the shore of your life have power. It is power to heal you of the need to generate life for others while forgetting to give birth to your own self.

In childbirth, by leaning into the pain, riding the waves of contractions, we work with our bodies to bring forth new life. All our instincts tell us to do otherwise. When we feel pain, we want to tense up, become rigid, and fight. Childbirth calls for us to become counterintuitive, coaching our bodies to work in tandem with the contractions as we prepare for giving birth.

During the rough storm of perimenopause, all your instincts will tell you to find ways to alleviate the symptoms; instead, become counterintuitive and work in tandem with the storm. Better yet, dive into the sea and ride its waves.

Jonathan Martin, in his poignant and beautiful book *How to Survive a Shipwreck*, describes what it is like to embrace the storm that seems bent on destroying your former life:

> These very waters that are drowning you now, have the life-giving power of Spirit within them, deep beneath the current. The waters that drag you down, where you do not wish to go—if you do not resist them—will spit you out like Jonah, spewed out of the belly of the whale. And you will burst out of the waters the second time, just like you did in the first—screaming in terror, shimmering in your sea-soaked, reddish new skin, glad to be out, terrified to be here . . . but damn here anyway, and so wonderfully alive, and breathing, and so terribly hopeful, no longer encumbered by unnecessary things like clothes, ideas, or expectations of what the world should be.[10]

The waves of perimenopause will drag you where you do not want to go. But for new life to emerge, you must lean into the pain, groaning and crying, all the while anticipating the new life waiting to burst forth. You must hold to the belief that the labor of perimenopause is giving birth to something wonderful—the part of you that was lost long ago. Your one precious self is in the deep, waiting to burst out of the waters just like she did the first time you were born.

Women in labor often choose to medicate through the roughest part of childbirth; you may choose to medicate during perimenopause. There is no harm in doing so, but do not medicate to the extent that you are numbed to the transformation going on inside you. Don't medicate to the point that you are unable to deal with repressed issues. Don't miss what is behind the door opened by this pain.

47

How do you lean into the storm? How do you work with the labor pains of perimenopause? *First, give yourself permission to open the door to the flood of repressed memories—anger, regret—as it begins to wash over you.* Ride these waves of remembering and see where they take you. What in those memories creates pain? What regrets do they contain? What things did you overlook for the sake of harmony that you are no longer willing to overlook?

Second, allow yourself to grieve what you lost. No one arrives at midlife without having suffered loss: jobs, husbands, parents, friendships, and even children. Perhaps at the time of loss you had the ability to move on, to put aside the grief for another day. Perhaps you were the kind of person who could put on a very good front, appearing as if nothing happened. Now, during this terrible storm, it may seem you are experiencing those events in fresh, painful ways. Guess what? Things did happen, and even if you brushed them aside, they never went away. They were stored in those deep caverns of your psyche. Now those memories are returning, and they are demanding your attention. Acknowledging them allows you to move into a new space—a space where you can come to terms with the depth of loss and pain rather than covering it up.

Third, enlist the support of other people. You may fear that in revisiting loss, pain, and disappointment you will become bogged down in the mire of it all and never get out. You are less likely to get lost in the pain if you enlist the help of a good therapist. A trained therapist, especially one who specializes in women's developmental issues, can help you interpret your feelings. A therapist offers a third-person perspective on your life. A person with this perspective often sees what you cannot see and in doing so gives you a new pair of eyes on events. A therapist also is able to give you the permission to lean into the storm when you can't give yourself permission.

Support groups are helpful for leaning into the storm. Sitting with other women who are also going through perimenopause helps you know you are not alone in the remembering, the anger, and the fear. Other women are experiencing the same things! But be careful in your choice of a support group. If you don't choose wisely, you may find yourself among a group of women intent on shutting down the process of uncovering. Women who have shut down their own process find special delight in "helping" others take the quick fix. "Just use essential oils" is not adequate advice for this phase of your life. Avoid women who overspiritualize your perimenopausal journey. "You need to pray about your anger issues" is a signal you need to run. You should also be careful to avoid a group composed of women whose experiences have them in complete disarray. A mass of drowning people can pull others down into the depths where they drown. Instead, look for a mixed group of women—those who are on the other side of menopause as well as those just entering this phase of life.

A supportive spouse is critical in reaping the benefits of the gift of uncovering. Your spouse does not have to understand what is happening to you, but it is important he give you the space to face this storm of deconstruction. If your husband attempts to rescue or protect you, he may cause the process to shut down before you are able to reap all the benefits of perimenopause. During the most difficult days of menopause, my husband, Jackie, was a steady, nonjudgmental presence. It was he who said, "This time of your life is difficult, but I believe it is a gift. After it's all over, why don't you write a book?"

Fourth, acknowledge that facing repressed issues puts you at risk for depression. During my perimenopausal journey, issues from growing up with a borderline narcissist mother resurfaced. At this time, my mother was aging, and she needed more care. But I had lived my entire life in fear of her. The tension between my fear of my mother and my desire to provide care for her pulled me down into a deep state of depression. I felt frozen, unable to think or act rationally. Thankfully, my physician ran what is called an integrated medicine clinic. His staff was trained to listen to women and to holistically guide them through menopause. In addition to compounded hormones, he prescribed Prozac. For about a year, this medication helped me in the journey through some deep anger and fear and prevented me from being overwhelmed with depression.

Fifth, allow yourself to ask the question "What if?" Midlife is a good time to revisit the choices you made, the deals you struck for the sake of harmony, and the missed opportunities. When you ask the question "What if?" you will find both the good and the bad. Yes, you will see the missed opportunities; you can grieve those. But you will also see how, at the time you made your decisions, you were doing the very best you could.

Sixth, face the ways in which others have taken advantage of your relational, pleasing self. During the first part of life, pleasing others may have been the mode you chose to maintain relationships. As Northrup explains, during our childbearing years, our biology works to encourage us to put the interests of others ahead of our own. She warns, "Culture's atmosphere of gender inequality exploits this tendency to an extreme."[11]

Perhaps people took advantage of your tendency to put the interests of others before your own. Perhaps you were passed over for promotion while others, less qualified than you, were praised and given promotions. Maybe your family expected you to work a full-time job and keep a perfect home. Perhaps your husband exploited your caring heart by having an affair and expecting you to get over it. Maybe word got out that you were "a nice woman," and people unloaded unreasonable demands on your time. Perhaps church leaders refused to use your gifts, all the while granting leadership to men who were less gifted and far less intelligent than you.

You will face a large amount of pent-up resentment as you see, perhaps for the first time, how much you sacrificed your own well-being for the sake of the well-being of others. Instead of damming up the anger and resentment, let it flow through you. Damming up these emotions is toxic! Go ahead, lean into the storm. Allow the waves of remembering to do their work—namely, to wash away the façade of the compliant, pleasing woman.

Seventh, forgive. Facing disappointments and regrets does not mean that you beat up on the younger version of yourself. As you face the resentment and anger, it is important to give yourself grace. Extend to yourself the same kindness you have always given to others. Forgive yourself for the decisions you regret.

You have to forgive not only yourself but also others. Choosing to forgive does not mean you pretend things did not happen. Rather, forgiveness means you choose not to allow the harm done to you by others to continue to have power over you. Forgiving and letting go is freeing. It moves you to a new place.

The practice of focused prayer is most helpful in facing the past, forgiving, and moving on. Focused prayer is not praying in order to gloss over events. Too many women think that prayer is a way of forgetting—as if by praying hard enough, the bad memories will go away. God does not forget the past. He redeems it. Unredeemed memories are like fresh wounds. Redeemed memories are like scars. They remind us of the wounds, but we no longer suffer from them.

During focused prayer, or healing prayer, you ask God to be present in the remembering of past injustice. During the remembering, the Holy Spirit will come alongside you, grieve with you and for you. If you surrender your pain to God, it is born by the wings of the Spirit into the presence of God, who redeems all things.

Forgiveness provides a space for your future to be born. It is a place of honesty and healing. Living in this place, you will not be the person of the past, the woman who was good at pretending or overlooking injustice to have harmony with others. Instead, you will become a person unwilling to overlook injustice. You will find yourself to be more outspoken and more assertive. Yet on the inside, you will be less judgmental and angry. People who are not in touch with their own feelings have a way of projecting those feelings onto others. People who are not in touch with their own hurt and anger are incapable of having empathy for the pain of others.

At some point during this journey, you will be tempted to believe that all the pain that comes from leaning into the storm is not worth it. There will come a point when you will begin to believe that you will be in the storm for the rest of your life. Believe me, the storm will pass. The calm will return. In the meantime, plunge into the deep, allowing the furious waves to destroy your too-small house. In *The Wizard of Oz*, Dorothy did not follow Aunt Em into the cellar. Instead, she rode the cyclone as it carried her far away from her small house in Kansas. After a while, she leaned in: "It was very dark, and wind howled terribly around her. . . . Hour after hour passed away, and slowly Dorothy got over her fright. At first she had wondered if she would be dashed to pieces when the house fell again; but as the hours passed . . . she stopped worrying and resolved to wait calmly and see what the future would bring."[12]

Get in Touch with Your Body

This may be hard to believe, but during the storm of perimenopause, your body can be your best friend. It may seem that your body is not your friend at all. It appears to be betraying you, plunging you into times of night sweats, tender breasts, heavy bleeding, and chronic fatigue. But your body is not betraying you; it is trying to help you let go of all the extra baggage you have forced it to carry around.

At this time of life, you have to trust your body, surrendering control over it in order to become present with it. Remember this: your body is not your enemy—it is your lifelong companion. Just as your body helped you navigate childhood and the radical changes of puberty and possibly childbirth, it will help you get through the rough terrain of perimenopause.

During perimenopause, your body is preparing for the changes necessary for the next phase of life. You have the choice of following its cues or resisting them. Trusting your body during the storm of perimenopause means that you believe it is taking you to a better place. It means you pay attention to the signals it sends about how to get to that better place. Let your body be your guide through the storm.

To trust your body, you first must learn to love it. Men find it easier to love their bodies than women. Some men seem to relish their expanding waistline, their graying hair, and the wrinkles on their face. It is as if these things make them wiser, seasoned, and more masculine. During faculty meetings, when my male colleagues want to make an important interjection, they often lean back and pat their stomach, as if by doing so they gain some greater wisdom. It is a strange irony—the larger the belly, the larger the self-confidence!

I never notice such behavior in women. The script we have been given tells us our bodies and our wisdom are forever disconnected. Our bodies are not our own; rather, they are the property of others. Early in life, we learn to give away our bodies to the judgment of others, the opinions of our friends, the images conveyed by media, the men in our lives, and the religious leaders intent on policing us. By midlife, we have learned that, when it comes to our bodies, there is always something in need of updating: thighs in need of toning, tummies in need of tucking, faces in need of injections, and hair in need of coloring. Skin needs to be sprayed a golden color. Eyelashes need extensions. Lips need plumping. Breasts need enlargement. Body renovation can easily become an obsession.

It is easy to see how women become obsessed with their aging bodies. We have inherited a long history of body shaming. Our foremothers were characterized as bent-over hags or toothless witches. Their bodies were viewed as useless as an old gray mare. During the Middle Ages, people believed that the bodies of post-menopausal women, due to the cessation of menstruation, be-came stagnant pools of "foul blood." These toxic bodies caused older women to become insane and unruly, with a tendency "to cause trouble." Parents were warned to keep their newborn babies away from postmenopausal hags lest their evil eyes put a curse on them.[13]

In seventeenth-century England, satires about the bodies of older women were popular. These poems showed contempt through exaggerated images of false teeth, hollow cheeks, and leather-like skin. The satirical poems of Puritan John Oldham were wildly popular. They were especially biting, describing older women as "lost and nasty souls" who were of such little value that they could be "hewn and cast down into the fire."[14] I will never forget the moment when presidential candidate Donald Trump called Hillary Clinton "such a nasty woman" during a televised debate. Listening to his words, I was horrified how the ancient image of older women as nasty continues to thrive.

I am grateful we live in an era that allows us women to age without losing all our teeth and having a face lined in wrinkles. Through exercise and diet, our bodies can look drastically different than those of our grandmothers. I have my grandparents' wedding picture, taken in 1905. My grandmother was in her mid-twenties, thin, and sporting a tiny waistline. I have a photo of her at seventy. Her gray hair is pulled back in a tight bun, and after giving birth to eleven children, her waistline has expanded to an extra-large size.

While modern women have greater opportunities to maintain healthy bodies, we continue to fear that one day we will become objects of ridicule. We know that our bodies are not our own— they must live up to the scrutiny of others. Women's bodies continue to be tied to sexuality and childbearing, but these two images are not allowed to exist together. In the Western world, small bodies are deemed more sexually attractive than larger ones. It is expected that women be eternally small and fertile. After giving birth, women are expected to shrink back into their prepregnancy size. If dieting and exercise don't work, we can always have plastic surgery to lose our mommy bodies. Women face the pressure of arriving at menopause with the body they developed in puberty: high breasts, small waist, and firm all over.

Here is our dilemma: at midlife, our minds may be full and our souls may be rich, but our bodies must be thin and firm. It is difficult to express our ideas, to speak our minds while living as fully embodied human beings. Cultural demands for thinness and hypersexuality cause us to disconnect our minds and our spirits from our bodies. Instead of viewing our bodies as a source of wisdom, they become a constant threat to our well-being. We are ever vigilant in keeping them in their proper place—our bodies become the enemy.

Northrup sees body acceptance as the final frontier for women. She notes that part of health at midlife is the ability to regain love for the body. The body, observes Northrup, is home to the soul. The body is the one thing that allows us to express our uniqueness on earth; we should cherish and listen to it.[15]

At perimenopause, your body seems to be betraying you; all the bodily symptoms are your body's way of begging you to no longer treat it like an enemy. It wants to reconnect with your soul. It wants to join back with you the way you were as a child—when your body expressed who you were and not just who you wanted to be.

Getting in touch with your body means taking note of the signals it sends without becoming obsessed with the physical symptoms themselves. You must train yourself to look beyond the symptoms to find the deeper messages they are sending you. As you enter perimenopause and experience the drop in progesterone, upsetting the estrogen-progesterone balance you have known for decades, your body will begin to adjust. During this time, you may experience heavy periods, breast tenderness, and fibroid tumors. Don't panic. Listen to your body's signals. They are telling you that the old pattern of living needs to change.

Perhaps you are the type of person who once could manage a great deal of stress, going without sleep and juggling several obligations. As you enter perimenopause, you will find it more difficult to be this person. Instead of thinking something is wrong with your body, look at your lifestyle. Your body is sending you signals that it is time to connect with it. Now is the time for uniting body and soul. Now is the time to listen to your body. It is not the time to force it into tight cultural molds. Love your body as it is.

Self-care during perimenopause is not something you do after you have tried everything else. It now becomes critical for overall well-being. There are some excellent books on the market right now that can help you in terms of learning the best foods, vitamins, and types of exercise for women going through the transition into menopause. Keep in mind that self-care is not the same as forcing your body into its earlier version.

Perimenopause is not the time to say, "I will honor my body by letting it go." While you shouldn't obsess over the shape and size of your body, you should pay attention to your physical health. Healthy bodies are related to healthy minds and souls. Depression and anxiety make it easy to neglect your body, so it is important to know about the snowball effect, which goes like this: I am depressed. To cope with my depression, I eat more junk food. Eating junk food causes me to gain a few extra pounds. With both depression and extra weight, exercise becomes more difficult. The less active I am, the more weight I gain. The more weight I gain, the more likely I am to develop type 2 diabetes, hypertension, and heart disease. If I develop any of these diseases, being an active person will be more difficult. The cycle continues until you become chronically ill, beset with a variety of problems.

Perimenopause and Early Life Trauma

I have known women who, once they started down the menopausal snowball-effect path, ended up on various medications for diabetes, hypertension, and heart disease. At some point, they passed the turning point, becoming unable to work and having to apply for disability benefits. Many of these precious women suffered abuse in childhood and spent most of their early adult years in bad relationships, low-wage jobs, and chronic economic distress. Over the course of time, these stressors exacted a heavy toll on their bodies. As they entered their midlife crisis, the perimenopause debt collector came and took everything. Their memories were too painful to bear. Their spirits were broken and their bodies worn-out.

It is becoming increasingly clear that early life stress can have long-lasting effects on parts of the brain responsible for emotions, mood, and memory. A recent study at the University of Pennsylvania concluded that women who suffered multiple traumatic events as they were growing up are at significant risk for perimenopausal depression.[16] In fact, women who experienced at least two adverse events during their formative years, whether abuse, neglect, or some type of family dysfunction, are more than twice as likely to experience depression during perimenopause.[17]

MARTHA

Martha grew up in a small Southern community. She was the oldest of four children, two girls and two boys. Their parents worked in a local cotton mill. Each evening their mother came home from the mill, cooked dinner, and cleaned the house. Martha and her sister helped with these tasks while their father and brothers spent time in the yard, fixing old cars and visiting with friends. Neither Martha's mother nor her father expended much energy on their children. They fed them, clothed them, and on occasion took them to church.

Martha and her sister were taught to be "nice girls." Being nice meant not talking too much, especially around men. Being nice meant taking the second seat in everything. It meant not speaking up for their own rights in order to favor the rights of others. Most of all, being nice meant living the lie that they did not matter. In Martha's culture, men were taught to look for a nice, pretty girl to marry. Marrying a nice, pretty girl was a ticket to ego strength and a life of affirmation of male superiority.

During work hours, Martha's mother left her children in the care of her sister. The sister's husband worked the night shift at the mill, so he was always at home when the children arrived. When Martha was twelve, her uncle began sexually abusing her. The abuse went on for four years, but Martha never spoke a word about it to her parents. She feared they would blame her. Her uncle told Martha that if she ever told anyone, he would do something really bad to her younger sister.

At sixteen, Martha quit school to marry her childhood sweetheart, Jerry. Martha's parents gave their permission for the marriage. They never considered how completing school might be more important than early marriage.

Jerry came from a troubled home. His mother was known in the community as the black sheep of her family, and Jerry grew up with serial fathers, some of whom were abusive to him and his mother. Most of Jerry's memories of the adults in his life involved heavy drinking and a great deal of violence. Jerry vowed to marry a nice girl, someone who was the opposite of his mother. He desperately wanted a normal wife and a normal life, but he had no idea what that would look like.

When Jerry met Martha, he knew she was different from his mother. She was extra nice, soft-spoken, and a very good girl. During their honeymoon, Martha told Jerry about her uncle's abuse. He went ballistic. "You are a whore, just like my mother!" he yelled. Jerry and Martha never again spoke of her sexual abuse, but their lives were colored by her shame and his anger.

Jerry longed for a normal life, but he did not know how to make it happen. He was driven by fear that one day everything would fall apart and his life would return to its former chaos. This fear caused him to become rigid and controlling, especially with those he loved.

Over the years, Jerry became extremely possessive of Martha. To keep her from having an affair, he would not allow her to work outside the home, except to clean houses and to sit with elderly people. He carefully vetted the families for whom Martha worked. All checks written for her work had to be in his name. The checking account, mortgage, and car loans were in Jerry's name alone. Although Martha knew how to drive, she rarely had cause to do so.

Martha's midlife crisis came when an eighteen-year-old teenager, Jackson, raped her sixteen-year-old daughter, Michelle. The rape occurred during a girls' sleepover at Jackson's house. Jackson's father was a dea-con of the church where Martha and Jerry were members. When her daughter confided in her about the rape, Martha tried to talk Jerry into confronting the young man and his family. He said he did not know what to do but suggested they talk with their pastor. During their conversation, Martha's pastor told her he would deal with the situation.

Eventually, during a time of prayer at church, the pastor's wife ap-proached Michelle and whispered into her ear, "God wants you to forgive Jackson. He is very sorry for what he did to you." The pastor's wife called the women of the church to gather around Michelle. Together, they prayed, asking God to give Michelle a spirit of forgiveness. Things were "settled," and everyone was expected to go on as if nothing had actually happened.

The rape and the way her church handled it so traumatized Michelle that she began to rebel against her father's strict rules and her church's double standard. She left home and began to take drugs. Michelle told her mother that all men were abusers and jerks. She vowed she would never walk through the doors of a church again.

Martha was furious about her daughter's rape and the church's treat-ment of her daughter, but she could not bring herself to openly express her anger. She knew doing so would incur the wrath of her husband, her extended family, and her church. Martha could not talk privately to her husband. By this time, he had concluded that their daughter had the same bad blood as his mother. He wanted nothing to do with Michelle.

During the next two years, Martha experienced the transition of peri-menopause. She was beset by waves of anger—anger at her husband for his controlling behavior, anger at her pastor and his wife for betray-ing her daughter. She began to remember her uncle's abuse and was shocked at the intensity of her memories. Even though he was dead, Martha fantasized about confronting him with a gun and shooting him, over and over. These thoughts both frightened Martha and gave her comfort.

Waves of anxiety followed on the heels of the anger. Martha became fearful that Michelle would die and go to hell. She became fearful that she was going to die and go to hell. Martha lost sleep, often spending the night walking the floors of the house and crying. During this time, she began calling her friends for support, keeping them on the phone for hours, pouring out a litany of anger and fear. Eventually, they stopped answering the phone. Martha's husband became more sullen and distant. He rarely spoke to her. He never touched her.

Martha's pain and anxiety eventually went underground into the only safe place it could find—her body. She began to suffer panic attacks. She gained a great deal of weight and was diagnosed with type 2 diabetes. Her knees became so bad that it was difficult for her to walk. Eventually, Martha was unable to work. Her outside outlets—housecleaning and elder care—were permanently closed. She stopped attending church, citing her health. She applied for disability and after several denials was granted the status of permanently disabled. Now Martha sleeps late. When she is awake, she numbs herself by watching continuous television. Martha is alone.

Women like Martha are more numerous than we realize. Multiple forms of stress, what psychologists define as complex trauma, characterize their lives. They have few external resources such as informed physicians, psychologists, and a supportive community. Their own internal resilience has never been developed. When the storm of perimenopause arrives, the hormonal changes triggering memory and anger only make things worse. In a desperate attempt at self-defense, the mind and the body begin to shut down, and these women experience a downward spiral that sometimes leads to an early death.

You may be a Martha. You may have experienced a great deal of trauma in your early life. You may currently be living in a situation characterized by abuse, control, and addictions. If so, don't despair. There are resources for you. *First, seek out a physician who sees you holistically and can help you read the signals your body is sending.* It is important to find a physician who is willing to go beyond prescribing medication to helping you find resources to cope with your trauma. Look for physicians who practice integrated medicine or holistic health.

Second, seek professional counseling, preferably with a therapist who specializes in trauma. I realize that therapy is costly and that most women cannot afford to pay for many sessions. Ask your physician if they can help you find a psychologist who counsels on a sliding scale that is based on income.

Third, if you are a victim of trauma, find good spiritual support. Seek out a wise pastor and look for a small group where you can safely share your feelings. It is deadly for traumatized women to be in a congregation that ties spiritual maturity to the ability to pretend nothing is wrong. Your lack of spirituality is not the problem. Your experience of trauma is what needs attention. You may have to leave your congregation in order to be part of a healing community, but know that your healing is worth the efforts to find another church.

Racial-Based Trauma and Generational Repercussions

Black women have longer and more difficult menopausal journeys than Caucasian women. A seventeen-year study of 1,449 women across the US found that, on average, women experienced menopausal symptoms for seven and a half years. However, the median length of time for black women was ten years. White women experienced symptoms for six and a half years. The study revealed that the menopausal journey of black women is not only longer but also more often filled with distressing symptoms such as hot flashes, depression, and anger.[18]

Black women not only have to contend with prejudice surrounding aging women but also have to bear the long legacy of racial trauma and its effects on their bodies. Writes Audre Lorde, "Ignoring the differences in race between women and the implications of those differences presents the most serious threat to mobilization of women's joint power."[19]

Postmenopausal power is joint power, and the perimenopausal storm is a shared storm. As we lean into this time of life, we should lean into the stories of all women and their ancestors.

Women of African descent in the United States have to contend with the horrific legacy of four hundred years of slavery, during which their foremothers endured unspeakable levels of terrorism, abuse, and rape. Enslaved women of African descent were used as sex slaves, and their wombs were viewed as commodities for breeding more slaves. Even after slavery ended, during the Jim Crow era, black women were portrayed as mammies and sexually aggressive Jezebels. This horrific legacy continues to bear its marks. Lisa Sharon Harper, founder and director of Freedom Road.us, observes, "A black woman's body is never her own. The oppression of black women takes multiple forms from childhood to menopause."[20]

During perimenopause, women remember past injustice. For many women of color, this process of remembering can be excruciating, especially when personal injustice is tied to corporate injustice. Harper began to research her family history. She discovered her great-great-great-grandmother, Lea, an enslaved woman whose body was used to bear her master seventeen children. Digging deeper, Harper discovered more stories of abuse and rape, some of which was perpetuated by members of her own family.

Perimenopause is the time to ask the question "What if?" Harper's "What if" questions flowed out of her family research: "What pathologies have state-enforced sexual violence caused within our families? How much healthier would we be if antebellum 'breeding' never happened? If family separation and loss never happened? If slavery never happened?"[21] You may ask, "What good does it do to drag up the past? Why not leave it buried?" The past is never really buried. It never goes away. Events happen, and memories of those events get coded into our brains. There those memories create their own world of genetic coding, one we pass down along generational lines.

Our Grandmother's Trauma

The emerging field of epigenetics, the study of biological mechanisms that switch genes on and off, offers clues as to how our grandmothers' traumas can become encoded in our own DNA. An article in the magazine *Discover* explains the epigenetic process:

> Like silt deposited on the cogs of a finely tuned machine after the seawater of a tsunami recedes, our experiences, and those of our forebears, are never gone, even if they have been forgotten. They become a part of us, a molecular residue holding fast to our genetic scaffolding. The DNA remains the same, but psychological and behavioral tendencies are inherited. You might have inherited not just your grandmother's knobby knees, but also her predisposition toward depression caused by the neglect she suffered as a newborn.[22]

Over the years, you may have swallowed your pain in huge toxic doses. Part of that pain may be some of your grandmother's. Perimenopause offers an opportunity to listen to your body as it tells you that it no longer wants your poison. It asks that you hear its cries and release it from the pain. There is new life on the other side.

The Benefits Outweigh the Pain

At first appearance, the gift of uncovering does not look anything like a gift. Its power to reveal the repressed and overlooked parts of our psyches can be terrifying. During my own journey, there were days when I feared the tears, the remembering, and the grief over the past would never go away. I feared the clouds of depression would never leave.

Looking back, I can see how I am in a much better place than before the storm. I am more aware of my reactions—my default response of fleeing the scene of distressing events. I am more aware of my tendency to agree to do things I don't want to do. I am more in touch with my limitations. I am more aware of the cumulative effect of generations of women in my family. I am more aware of my residual fear of sharp criticism and harsh words and my own tendency to blame the victim.

Because of the storm of perimenopause, I am more aware of how my body keeps score. I have learned to pay attention to the signals it sends when I am under stress or going through trauma. The gift of uncovering has helped me get in touch with the hidden recesses of my psyche—what Carl Jung refers to as the shadow side. Knowing the shadow side, those parts of myself I want to keep hidden, helps me live with a more sober vision of myself. I am not perfect. I have limitations.

Refusing the gift of uncovering means you will have more difficulty facing second-half-of-life tasks. Resistance means you will continue to be burdened with baggage from the past, baggage that will make it extremely difficult for you to set your sails for unchartered waters. You have the choice—open the door and let the winds blow you into a new place or batten down the hatches, huddle in a dark corner, and ride out the storm. Choose wisely.

Personal Reflection Activities

1. What words would you use to describe your experience of perimenopause?

2. How has the bill collector come calling?

   What are the things you are paying attention to that you once overlooked?

   What things that you believed were long forgotten are now bubbling to the surface?

3. In what ways do you feel out of control? What are your fears?

4. Using the suggestions given in this chapter, write your own personal plan of leaning into the storm of perimenopause.

5. If you have experienced trauma in your life, list the steps you will take to get help in dealing with the flood of painful memories you may be experiencing.

   What physician specializing in holistic medicine is available in your area?

   How can you locate a therapist or counselor specializing in trauma?

   What support groups are available in your area?

   What type of church do you need right now?

   What do you need from your spouse?

   What people or places do you need to avoid at this time in your life?

   Who do you need to forgive?

Group Reflection Activities

1. Take a few minutes (no more than five minutes for each person) for anyone in your group to share her experiences of the storm of perimenopause and the gift of uncovering.

2. What common themes do you see emerging from the time of sharing? List these themes for everyone to see.

3. Ask the following questions:

   What do we all have in common?

   What is unique about each person's experience? How do issues such as culture and ethnicity factor into our experiences?

THREE

THE GIFT
OF ANGER

You should be angry. . . . Use that anger. You write it. You paint it.
You dance it. You march it. You vote it. You do everything about
it. You talk it. Never stop talking it.

—Maya Angelou, from an interview with Dave Chappelle

HIDDEN WITHIN THE GIFT of uncovering is another gift: anger. This
gift arrives in various forms, ranging from a diffused and gener-
alized sense of anger to intense, overwhelming episodes of what
is known as perimenopausal rage. The anger women experience
at perimenopause happens when estrogen and its lovely dance
companion, serotonin, are out of sync. While these two mood
regulators work to rebalance themselves, the part of the brain that
triggers anger awakens from its slumber. It has been hidden since
adolescence, kept under control by a potent stew of hormones.
With the stew of hormones dissipating at perimenopause, anger
seizes its chance to make itself known. "Free at last! Free at last!"
is the mantra of perimenopausal anger.

Anger's arrival takes most women by surprise. The anger mechanism has been dormant for so long that most women have forgotten it exists. Oh, it does exist, and it returns with attitude. For too long, anger has bent to our will to overlook injustice, to let offenses go for the sake of relational harmony. The force of anger takes things that have been simmering on the back burner of our psyches and brings them to the front, where the heat is turned up. Long forgotten memories begins to boil.

The boiling pot of anger on the front burner of our psyches signals that now is the best time to come to terms with repressed anger. Writes Christiane Northrup, "If, before menopause, a woman hasn't learned to identify her anger and what it is telling her (and this describes many women), perimenopause is her best remaining opportunity to do so."[1] Perimenopause gives us this window of opportunity by rewiring the brain in a way that helps us see things clearer. For the first time in decades, we are able to see our own anger.

Of all the gifts of menopause, anger is the most misunderstood. In fact, most women believe that anger is not a gift at all; it is a defect of character, something to be avoided. Some would even venture to say that the words *anger* and *women* don't belong in the same sentence. The assumption has long been that angry women have no place in the world.

Historically, anger has been the domain of men. It is expected that men will show their anger, and they are given a great deal of latitude in ways of expressing it: raising their voice, writing an op-ed piece, slamming their fist on the table, or simply saying, "You have made me angry!" Angry men have dueled, fought in fistfights, and gone on killing sprees with their AK-15s in hand. In some cultures, it is permissible for men to show anger by hitting women. "I should not have made him angry" is an all-too-common phrase I have heard from battered women.

When it comes to women, anger is a forbidden fruit. In a 2010 large-scale study conducted in the US and Canada, only 6.2 percent of people thought that expressing anger is appropriate for women.[2] This statistic is staggering; it means that 93.8 percent of respondents believed it is inappropriate to be an angry woman.

Women fear anger, especially the intense perimenopausal rage that leaves us feeling ashamed of our outbursts. We fear anger the same way we fear our bodies, and we treat anger the same way we treat our bodies. We believe that something is inherently wrong with both. We are hypervigilant, ever aware of the appearance of our bodies. We closely monitor our anger believing that it can easily spin out of control. Sadly, we view our bodies and our anger as unfamiliar and hostile spaces.

Harriet Lerner points out that women fear anger not only because it brings about the disapproval of others but also because it signals the necessity for change. We cannot mature into the second half of life without change, and sometimes we have to get angry enough to change things. Lerner notes that anger is neither legitimate nor illegitimate. It simply is. She writes, "To ask, 'do I have a right to be angry' is like asking, 'do I have a right to be thirsty?'"[3] Perimenopausal anger is like the thirst during a long walk in the desert; it is demanding and incessant. You don't have this anger—it has you!

"Anger is a sign that you've been putting up with things that haven't served you fully—and you're not willing to put up with them anymore," writes Northrup. At midlife, we feel a fierce need to "have our say and to be heard—sometimes for the first time in decades. Many of us stifled our true voice sometime in adolescence, when we were more concerned with fitting in, finding our place, and following the rules."[4]

From adolescence onward, women not only work hard to stifle anger but also become adept at deflecting it. "Oh, I'm not angry.

I'm disappointed." "Oh no, you're mistaken. I'm not angry. I'm just hurt." Here is my favorite deflection: "I'm not angry, just thinking." It is a good thing that perimenopausal anger arrives with such intensity!

We deflect anger because we know it is not welcome. It is not welcome in churches or civic groups. It is not welcome on the internet. We all know the caricatures: the angry bitch or the harassing nag. Women are allowed to be hurt. We are allowed to cry. Millions of angry tears have been shed in the name of "being hurt."

Because we live in a world where women's anger is not welcome, we have to work extra hard to claim this gift. Once claimed, anger can be channeled into a creative force, one that has the power to propel us into a healthier and more authentic way of existence.

Anger is a human right, and as a human right, it is the right of women. In her book *Rage Becomes Her*, Soraya Chemaly gives a full and accurate description of anger:

> Anger is an assertion of rights and worth. It is communication, equality, and knowledge. It is intimacy, acceptance, fearlessness, embodiment, revolt, and reconciliation. Anger is memory and rage. It is rational thought and irrational pain. Anger is freedom, independence, expansiveness, and entitlement. It is justice, passion, clarity, and motivation. Anger is instrumental, thoughtful, complicated, and resolved. In anger, whether you like it or not, there is truth. Anger is the demand of accountability. It is evaluation, judgment, and refutation. It is reflective, visionary, and participatory. It's a speech act, a social statement, an intention, and a purpose. It's risk and threat. A confirmation and a wish.
>
> It is both powerlessness and power, palliative and a provocation. In anger, you find both ferocity and comfort, vulnerability and hurt. Anger is the expression of hope.[5]

Anger and "the Nice Lady Syndrome"

Anger is a life force. It is a cleansing fire; when used properly, it makes way for much of life's dead wood to be cleared out so new growth can occur. If handled wrongly, anger's power becomes a raging wildfire, destroying everything in its path, including the person who is angry.

Women are adept not only at deflecting anger but also at masking it. Masking anger is one of the most common and unhealthy ways of dealing with anger. Women mask anger with what Harriet Lerner describes as "the nice lady syndrome."[6] You know the nice lady. She is the person people call on to get things done at the last minute. She is the person who never complains, never gets angry, and is always smiling.

The nice lady's voice is forever pitched upward into a sunny singsong cadence. She is the woman who answers her phone with an upward lilt: "This is Sue. How can I help you?" By the time she says the last word—*you*—her voice is two octaves higher than when she began the sentence.

There is an irony to being the nice lady. On the surface, a nice lady appears passive and easy to get along with. In actuality, a woman expends a great deal of energy being nice. Lerner points out that nice ladies have "developed an important and complex interpersonal skill that requires a great deal of our inner activity and sensitivity." Nice ladies "are good at anticipating other people's reaction. . . . They are experts at protecting others from uncomfortable feelings."[7] Being the nice lady is a complex social skill requiring a great deal of intuitive energy. It is exhausting being the nice lady.

We often believe the nice lady never gets angry. That is where we are wrong. Her anger is there, but it is woven so tightly within the fabric of her persona that she is unable to access her own feelings. Being the nice lady requires a woman to disconnect from her own psyche. Too much of her energy is invested in reading and responding to the signals of others. There is no room to read her own signals. The nice lady rarely knows if she is angry, sad, or even deeply hurt. The nice lady knows that accessing the anger or other deep feelings would destroy the persona she has worked since puberty to construct.

If you are serious about reaping the benefits of the gift of anger, the place to begin is with a self-analysis of the strength of your inclination to play the nice lady role. Are you programmed to respond to external cues at the expense of your own thoughts? Are you prone to ignore your own ideas and go along with the ideas of others? Do you live on high alert, ready to respond to the demands of others? Do you work hard to diffuse the anger of your spouse—even at the expense of your own integrity? Do you allow others to take advantage of you, all the while seething inside?

Women's Health and Repressed Anger

If you have been on the giving end of relationships to the extent that you have lost a sense of your own power and identity, be prepared to experience the effects of repressed anger. The anger can show up masked within physical symptoms such as migraine headaches, fibroid tumors, and diseases such as fibromyalgia. Anger not expressed can also show up in depression.

Too many women rush for treatment of the physical symptoms of perimenopause without stopping to reflect on their deeper needs. If you are having episodes of perimenopausal rage, moments of uncontrolled anger, you will need some extra help. You may need medication such as hormone therapy or antidepressants.

But be careful not to overmedicate to the point that you lose touch with your anger.

The best way to understand how anger is affecting your health is to get in touch with your emotions. Emotions are our inner guidance system. They are not signs of weakness. Women are not overemotional. We are fully embodied people, artfully woven masterpieces of mind, emotions, and will. During perimenopause, our emotions serve as our friends. They are the messengers signaling how we need to change our old ways of being in the world. Writes Northrup, "Understanding how your thoughts and your emotions affect every single hormone and cell in your body, and how to change them in a way that is health-enhancing, gives you access to the most powerful and empowering health-creating secret on earth."[8]

Linking anger to our health helps us see how important it is that we pay attention to the mind-body connection. Emotions help us pay attention to our anger, but anger is not merely an emotion. It is a whole body experience, one that is hardwired into our autonomic nervous system. The autonomic nervous system is divided into two parts: the parasympathetic nervous system and the sympathetic nervous system. These two systems work together in regulating the organs in our bodies.

Northrup describes the parasympathetic nervous system (PNS) as the brake in the body. She writes, "It promotes functions associated with growth and restoration, rest and relaxation, and deals primarily with conservation of body energy by causing your vital organs to 'rest' when they are not on duty."[9] The sympathetic nervous system (SNS) functions as the gas of the body's systems. Describes Northrup, "It revs up your metabolism to deal with challenges from outside the body. Stimulation of the SNS quickly mobilizes your body's reserves so that you can protect and defend yourself."[10] The SNS causes the fight-or-flight mechanism to kick in. The SNS sends the message, "Prepare for battle." In response, our eyes dilate and our blood vessels constrict, causing blood pressure to rise. Blood is borrowed from the intestinal reservoir and shunted to major muscles, lungs, heart, and brain.

Far too many women live in a constant state of agitation. Beneath the calm surface, their sympathetic nervous system is working overtime. Their parasympathetic system rarely gets a chance to do its job of restoring and resting the body's vital systems. Years of living on high alert take their toll on the body.

Perimenopausal anger is the body's wake-up call, alerting us to the need to pay attention to the toll repressed anger is taking on our bodies. What lies beneath is active, coursing through the systems of our bodies, even when we are not conscious of its presence. Pay attention to your body's signals. Respond proactively: let the anger come to the surface, then seek healing.

RENITA

After graduating from university, Renita went to work as an assistant for a program director of a Christian organization. Although she was overqualified for the position, Renita told herself that the job would provide income until she found a better position. Ten years later, Renita was still in this "temporary" job. In the interim, she had trained two bosses, both of whom had the same level of education as she.

Hoping to advance within the institution, Renita took advantage of online education and earned an MBA. No one seemed to notice. When positions became available, Renita applied for them, hoping she would be chosen. Each time the organization hired a male less qualified than Renita.

Ten years turned into twenty, and Renita, now in her late forties, still has the same job she began right after university. During her perimenopausal storm, Renita has become skillful at channeling her anger at the

76

organization in passive-aggressive ways. When she is in the office, she is sullen, intentionally making mistakes she knows will make the organization look bad.

Over the years, Renita's health has declined. She misses more and more work due to constant migraines. She has gained forty pounds; she doesn't exercise or eat well. Every evening Renita comes home from work, fixes dinner, and goes to the couch, where she binge watches television. Before she goes to sleep, Renita recalls all the offenses leveled against her during the day. She complains to her husband about the lack of opportunities within the organization. The next day she arrives at work and goes through the same routine: sullen behavior, biting remarks to people, intentional mistakes in her work.

Perimenopause offers Renita an opportunity to get in touch with her anger and to reassess where she is in life. It offers an open door for Renita to find a new level of self-direction and assertiveness. But Renita was groomed to behave otherwise. She is part of a religious tradition that labels assertive women as "radical feminists."

Not wanting to be one of those radical women, Renita internalized the narrative given to her. It is a script telling her that if she would be a good girl, eventually someone would recognize her gifts and make space for them. After years of disappointment, after decades of being a good girl, her confidence has eroded to the degree that she is codependent on a system that treats her as an inferior person.

Women like Renita often lack the ability to find and use anger as a guide for self-discovery. What would happen if Renita began to own her anger? How could she allow this anger to guide her toward a new way of being in the world? What if she allowed her anger to propel her into a new space in life? You may be a Renita. If so, it is time to claim the gift of anger.

The Rise of Women's Corporate Anger

Anger is a force that propels us into new life as individuals. Anger is also a force with the power to propel societies into new life. Women's anger is now a major social force in American society.

#MeToo

The #MeToo movement was started by a black woman and social activist named Tarana Burke. In 2006, Burke began using the phrase "Me Too" to raise consciousness of the pervasiveness of sexual abuse and assault in society. In 2017, the phrase became part of a broader movement of women's anger. This broader movement began with a series of shattering articles published in the *New York Times* and the *New Yorker* regarding movie producer Harvey Weinstein and his decades-long history of sexual harassment, abuse, and alleged rape of young actresses. Following the Weinstein revelations, on October 15, 2017, actress Alyssa Milano tweeted, "If you've been sexually harassed or assaulted, write 'me too' as a reply to this tweet." Milano's tweet opened a floodgate of responses.

In addition to the Weinstein revelations, allegations against R. Kelly—a singer, songwriter, and music producer—began to surface. Dating as far back as 1992, these allegations tell the story of rape, abuse, and holding adult women against their will. The documentary *Surviving R. Kelly* made it impossible for the well-established pattern of Kelly's abuse to remain hidden.

Over the next few months, millions of women tweeted, wrote Facebook posts, blogged, and published op-ed articles narrating their experiences of sexual harassment. I remember reading these accounts with both great sadness and great horror. These stories were filled with accounts of emotional trauma, physical violence, and professional losses. They told the hard truth about cover-up, silencing, and blaming the victim. Older women, some in their seventies and eighties, for the first time in their lives dared to share long-repressed trauma involving childhood abuse and sexual harassment in the workplace.

During this time when women's hidden stories were being revealed, I had a conversation with Margaret, a seventy-five-year-old woman, after our water aerobics class. As we sat in the hot tub at the YMCA, she told me her story of being in the military, where she was the only woman training men in technical aspects of airplane instrument reading. "I was respected. I loved my job. But a new supervisor came into my department." Margaret went on to describe how shortly after arriving, the man approached her, making it clear that if she wanted to continue her position, there would be a certain price to pay.

Margaret proudly smiled as she told me how she went above rank and, in a subtle way, asked her commanding officer, "What could one do if they were being pressured to do things with which they were uncomfortable?" She told me how the officer responded with, "Don't you worry. Let me take care of things." The supervisor was removed, and Margaret continued her job. Women needed to "play it cool" and "not be too direct," she told me.

As Margaret offered her advice, I could not help thinking of how lucky she was that her commanding officer picked up on her subtle request. What if he had not done so? There are certainly plenty of women who may have been ignored or even punished for coming forward under similar circumstances. I can understand how Margaret formed her opinion that one needed to play it cool and take the indirect approach. Women of her generation had no personal power. Direct confrontation was impossible, making subtlety the only way forward.

#ChurchToo

On November 20, 2017, Emily Joy shared on Twitter her story of being groomed and abused ten years earlier: "When I was 16 years old I was groomed for abuse by a man in his early 30s who was a 'youth leader' in my evangelical megachurch, Northwoods Community Church in Peoria, IL." Immediately, women, both old and young, responded with their own stories of abuse by church leaders. A few days later, the hashtag #ChurchToo was born.

The #ChurchToo movement spread quickly. It ignited Facebook groups and conferences and was the subject of many blog posts and Christian magazine articles.[11] In December 2018, Wheaton College, the flagship of evangelical higher education, sponsored a conference on the topic of abuse in the church. At this conference, evangelical leaders such as Max Lucado and Beth Moore revealed their own stories of abuse.[12]

In response to both the #MeToo movement and the #ChurchToo movement, authors and activists Belinda Bauman and Lisa Sharon Harper created #SilenceIsNotSpiritual. They gathered thousands of signatures in support of a statement that reads in part, "This moment in history is ours to steward. We are calling churches . . . to end the silence and stop all participation in violence against women. We call our pastors, our elders, and our parishioners who have been silent to speak up and stand up for all who experience abuse. There is no institution with greater capacity to create protected spaces for healing and restoration for survivors, as well as confession, repentance and rehabilitation for perpetrators."[13]

At this time in your life, you may be reliving painful memories of abuse. Your abuse may have occurred at the hands of a spiritual leader. It may have taken place within the sacred grounds of a church. To make matters worse, your cries for justice may have been silenced—by your parents, church leaders, and even your own shame. Know that you are not alone and know also that there is a God who sees (Gen. 16:13).

I have been drawn to explore a couple of passages of terror in the Old Testament: the rape and murder of the unnamed concubine (Judg. 19) and the rape of Tamar, the daughter of King David (2 Sam. 13:1–22). In both texts, the question "Where was God?" begs to be answered. I believe God's presence is found in the grieving Spirit of *Shekinah*. In Jewish tradition, *Shekinah* offers an image of God's willed presence, a presence that assumes feminine form. *Shekinah* is the one who goes with Israel into hostile territory. "When the people are brought low then *Shekinah* lies in the dust, anguished by human suffering."[14]

It is helpful to know that *Shekinah* was present in the concubine's journey. She was present in the house of David. When the Levite opened the door and found his concubine lying in the dust at the doorstep, *Shekinah*—the willed presence of God—was lying in the dust with her. When Tamar ran from her brother's chamber, tearing her garments, throwing ashes over her head, *Shekinah*—the willed presence of God—was there with her.

We often assume that God is distant, someone looking down on our suffering but not participating in our pain. Nothing could be further from the truth. God's Spirit is actively involved in creation: grieving over the brokenness, brooding over the chaos, and working to transform everything that has been marred by sin. In the incarnation, Jesus became flesh—fully divine and fully human. He suffered torture and execution. He endured loneliness and abandonment. His loud cries in the Garden of Gethsemane went unnoticed by his closest friends.

Women who have suffered in church settings are not abandoned to grief. God's Spirit is at work toward justice and healing. We can join in this work by vowing that we will no longer keep silent in the face of injustice and abuse. In the era of #MeToo and #ChurchToo, we can pray the words of ancient Syriac Christians: "Holy Spirit, merciful mother, spread your wings over our sinful times."[15] There will be a time for the fullness of the new order of creation. Until then, the Holy Spirit broods and hovers over her work.

How to Claim the Gift of Anger

Understand Anger as Power

While most women will agree that repressed anger can be both a physical and a mental health hazard, it is hard for us to channel our anger in a life-giving manner. One of the main reasons we are so angry is that we feel powerless. Understanding anger as power is a necessary first step in claiming the gift of anger. In her essay "The Uses of Anger," Audre Lorde describes this power: "Every woman has a well-stocked arsenal of anger potentially useful against those oppressions, personal and institutional, which brought that anger into being. Focused with precision it can become a powerful source of energy serving progress and change. And when I speak of change, I do not mean a simple switch of positions or a temporary lessening of tensions, nor the ability to smile or feel good. I am speaking of a basic and radical alteration in those assumptions underlining our lives."[16]

Lorde is speaking primarily to black women, but all women need to hear her voice. Anger is an intersectional issue, crossing the lines of ethnicity, class, and education level. There are many significant voices coming from women of color—voices such as that of Austin Channing Brown, whose book *I'm Still Here: Black Dignity in a World Made for Whiteness* reveals the daily microaggressions black women endure, even in organizations that claim to be free of racial bias.[17]

The angry black woman trope makes it especially difficult for black women to express anger. If they show anger, white people respond, "She sure has an attitude!" Writes Brown, "Instead of anger, I would try to communicate other emotions that I thought might receive an audience—pain, disappointment, sadness. I would roll up my sleeves and reveal the scars, cut myself open and hope that the blood that emerged would move my listeners."[18] Brown realized that instead of expressing her anger, she was working not to be destroyed by her own rage. By reading the writings of people such as Lorde, Brown was liberated. She writes, "Anger is not inherently destructive. My anger can be a force for good. My anger can be creative and imaginative, seeing a better world that doesn't yet exist. It can fuel a righteous movement toward justice and freedom. I don't need to fear my own anger."[19]

Develop Anger Competency

The second step in claiming the gift of anger is to develop what Soraya Chemaly calls "anger competency."[20] I like the phrase "anger competency" much better than "anger management." Anger management techniques seek to rein anger in, but anger is not limited to being a negative and destructive emotion.

One of the ways to gain anger competency is by developing self-awareness. The storm of perimenopause can be a force that reveals hidden aspects of your personality. As you lean into this storm, take time to probe your anger, taking stock of your choices, behavior, and how you manage your relationships. Chemaly recommends that you take stock of your default anger settings. She writes, "Are you expressive or a ruminator? Do you simmer or explode? Do you cry or calmly assert yourself? Are you diverting your anger? Do you even admit to yourself that you are mad about something or at someone close to you?"[21]

During my perimenopausal storm, my therapist talked with me about what she called my default buttons. Our default buttons are the way we were programmed by our family of origin to respond to stress. I discovered how, as the oldest child, I was programmed to try to calm the anger of others. "Being good" was a way of keeping my mother's rage at bay. Another default button was to run away and ruminate on the things that made me angry. Expressing anger openly was dangerous, so I took it outside into the woods, where I would spend hours alone, daydreaming of escape.

Journaling can also help you develop anger competency. Remember the diary you kept during puberty and how it was a safe place to channel your angst, fears, and desires? Journaling is a helpful practice during perimenopause. It allows you to make external what you are feeling inside. It helps you objectify the world, muse on events, and reflect on your feelings without pausing to think about how your words will be received by others. Your journal can be a place where you write letters that you don't intend to mail. Writing letters to people who hurt you in the past allows you to face them again and express what the earlier, nice version of yourself failed to express. Write letters to yourself. Looking back, what would you say to the twenty-year-old who had just fallen in love with the man of her dreams? What would you say to the young woman who allowed others to take advantage of her time?

As you fill in the pages of your journal and express yourself in unmailed letters, your anger will guide you through the most difficult times. Keep telling yourself that in expressing the anger you are giving voice to the hidden parts of you. Your voice, no matter the anger or hurt it expresses, needs to have space to speak.

Expressing your anger to others in clear and nonthreatening ways is another way to develop anger competency. As much as you journal or write letters, there will be times when you need to express your anger to others. You will need to do this to redefine the terms of your relationships and find healing. It is important to express anger to others in clear, non-blaming ways. When you write a letter, it will not push back. Talking with people will garner a response.

Before talking with others about your anger, take stock of your words. How often do you use the blaming language of "you"? Use of the pronoun "you" makes others defensive; on the other hand, the pronoun "I" is less threatening. Learn to replace sentences such as "You never help me around the house" with "I feel overwhelmed with all the responsibilities right now. I need help."

As you begin to express your anger, be prepared for pushback from those closest to you. We do not live in isolation. All of us exist in larger systems, such as families and places of employment. These systems function when everyone fulfills his or her role, but when one member of the system changes, the entire system gets out of balance. Disequilibrium is met with resistance.

It is normal for people within a system to want to keep it going in ways that have worked before. As already noted, the people in your life want you to return to the person they knew before you entered the storm of perimenopause. However, you now realize how these systems have worked at your expense. But be careful to avoid playing the victim. Don't become the drama queen. Instead, use your anger to find your voice.

When the pushback comes, stand your ground and speak using clear, non-blaming statements regarding your expectations. Again, use the pronoun "I" instead of "you." "I feel that I am often taken advantage of" is better than "You often take advantage of me." By using "I," you are more likely to be heard.

Learning to distinguish between anger, assertiveness, and aggression can also help you develop anger competency. Chemaly writes, "Anger, assertiveness, and aggression are frequently and unhelpfully lumped together, particularly when the person who is being assertive, angry or aggressive is a girl or woman."[22] She notes that assertiveness is the act of stating a position with confidence. Assertiveness involves direct, clear, and honest communication. "Assertive women are more emotionally silent and less likely to experience anxiety or depression."[23]

Aggression is more confrontational behavior. The root of the word *aggressive* is related to the Latin word *aggredi*, meaning "to go forward." Aggression can be less civil, but as Chemaly points out, it can be respectful. "It is possible to be both assertive and aggressive without being angry at all, and conversely, to be angry without being assertive or aggressive."[24]

In recent years, I have noticed that I don't have a problem being assertive. Usually, I am able to state my opinion on most matters and to do so clearly. What I do have a problem with is being aggressive. Receiving pushback causes me to yield the right-of-way to others. After yielding, I hate myself for giving in to the plans of others so quickly. Externally I am compliant, but internally I am screaming questions at myself: "Why didn't you stand your ground? Why didn't you stand up for yourself?" I have come to realize that as much as I call myself a feminist, deep down I believe that when push comes to shove, women are supposed to yield. This revelation has been sobering, and I am determined to be more aggressive.

Not long ago, I had a test of my resolve. I teach a doctorate-level course that meets every third Friday. We meet in an assigned room. Unknown to me, a couple of my colleagues were using the room for a class that meets once a month. On the scheduled day of my class, I walked in to find my two male colleagues setting up for their class. I told them that my class meets in this location every three weeks and that the room had been assigned by the dean's office. They did not believe me, stating, "We have met here every month." I responded that the times they met in the room had not overlapped with mine until this particular day.

My colleagues were unimpressed with my explanation and continued to set up their laptops. I assumed an aggressive posture with both feet firmly planted on the floor. With direct eye contact, I spoke in a clear, deep voice. "I am not leaving. You will have to make other arrangements." After a few moments of silence, the guys got my message and found another location for their class.

The old me would have yielded the room. "Oh, no problem. Since you guys were already here, I will find another room." The old me would have left the room seething with anger, asking myself, "Why do you always give in?" The new, more aggressive me stood her ground and claimed the room. That morning I discovered how aggressiveness saved me from being angry. Standing my ground kept me from being angry with my colleagues, and I was not angry with myself for yielding to them. I was merely claiming my room.

As already mentioned, the angry black woman trope makes it difficult for black women to express their anger. It is also difficult for black women to be assertive or aggressive. A black woman who is being assertive or aggressive is not seen in the same way as a white woman who behaves the same way. Over the years, I have heard white people complain about black women not knowing their place. Black women are more often described as pushy and bossy when they are just standing their ground.

Women who live in conservative, patriarchal environments have an especially hard time owning their anger. In their world, even basic self-expression is viewed with disdain. Just daring to speak and share your opinion on a matter may be hazardous. If you are a woman who lives in such an environment, you will need extra support to show your anger. You will need safe places. Consider the cost of expressing your anger, and do your very best to be true to yourself.

Anger is a powerful, creative emotion. It is helpful in moving us to action. But I have learned that far too often a woman's default mode is to avoid assertiveness and aggression. Work on being more assertive. You will find that in doing so you will have less hidden anger. Work on being more aggressive. In doing so, you will notice that your life energy is clearing a path for you to move forward.

Place Your Anger within the Larger Movement of Women's Anger

When we are going through our own season of anger, it is difficult to see beyond our own maelstrom. After all, we are the one going through the remembering, the pain. It is up to each of us to develop anger competency. Yet the gift of anger is not completely individualized and separate from the experiences of other women.

Women's anger can be a cacophony of disparate, individual voices, or it can be a symphony of harmonized energy. Each of us has our unique voice of anger. The sound of our anger, joined with that of others, has the power to create new ways of being human.

As a Christian, I believe God's Spirit is at work among women. Just as the wind of God swept over the primal waters, generating life, God's Spirit is sweeping over women, stirring up the waters of our anger. Beneath those waters a new world is waiting to emerge—a world where women are free to creatively channel their anger for the causes of justice. It is a world where our daughters will grow up never feeling the need to swallow their anger or to deflect it. It is a world where the nice ladies are rare and powerful women are common.

Take stock of your anger and look around. Where do you see other women expressing their anger? How can you join with them in addressing issues such as abuse, injustice, and human trafficking? We are women. Hear us roar.

Looking Ahead

"Perimenopausal anger," writes Christiane Northrup, is "the energy needed to propel you into your new life." She goes on to say, "If the symptoms of perimenopause are the labor pains we experience as we give birth to our authentic selves at midlife, then our anger is the cry of our newborn selves whom we've just birthed."[25]

Your anger is the signal that another gift is about to be born—the gift of the authentic self. Trust me, you will love her.

Personal Reflection Activities

1. Take a moment to describe the messages you grew up with about women's anger. After writing, ask yourself, "How have I internalized the messages I received about women's anger?"
2. On a scale of 1 to 10, with 1 being the lowest and 10 being the highest, how would you rate the intensity of your anger?
3. In what ways have you internalized the images of the nice lady? Describe what sacrifices you have made to assume this role.
4. Do you experience episodes of perimenopausal rage? If you do, describe these episodes.
   What triggers them?
   How do you feel in the midst of the rage?
   How do you feel after the rage has passed?

Develop a plan for proactively addressing these episodes. You may consider the following:

Schedule an appointment with your physician to discuss these episodes.
Consider hormone therapy.
Consider other medication, such as antidepressants.
Seek out a therapist competent in women's anger.

5. Using the suggestions given in this chapter, write your own personal plan for developing anger competency.

Group Reflection Activities

1. Take a few minutes to discuss the stereotypes of angry women. Ask, "How have we internalized these images?"
2. Talk about your reactions to abuses such as those highlighted in the discussion about the #MeToo and #ChurchToo movements.

   What memories have these accounts brought to the surface?
   How can we relate our personal stories of anger with those of other women?

3. As a group, discuss ways to develop anger competency.

   What steps are the hardest to accomplish?
   What keeps you from creatively channeling your anger?

4. End the session by speaking a blessing over women's anger.

FOUR

THE GIFT
OF THE
AUTHENTIC SELF

The most common form of despair is not being who you are.

—Søren Kierkegaard, *The Sickness Unto Death*

Our deepest calling is to grow into our own authentic self-hood, whether or not it conforms to some image of who we ought to be.

—Parker Palmer, "Now I Become Myself" in *Yes! Magazine*

Some women get erased a little at a time, some all at once Some reappear. Every woman who appears wrestles with the forces that would have her disappear. She struggles with the forces that would tell her story for her, or write her out of the story, the genealogy, the rights of man, the rule of law. The ability to tell your own story, in words or images, is already a victory, already a revolt.

—Rebecca Solnit, *Men Explain Things to Me*

WANEDA BROWNLOW

At the age of fifty, Waneda lived a full and contented life. She was a well-educated woman who spoke three languages. She regularly traveled to exotic places in the world. She worked as a missionary alongside her husband for many years. They served in Italy, Guatemala, Russia, and Belize.

After several years abroad, Waneda and her husband returned to the United States. Waneda had a degree in elementary education, so she began to teach in public schools. Through the years, she enjoyed teaching and the perks of having her summers free to be with her family. In midlife, it seemed that Waneda's life would continue much as it had been in previous years. Other than dreams of retirement, neither she nor her husband had plans for dramatic changes.

Waneda's world was shattered when her husband died suddenly from a massive heart attack. To make matters worse, while grieving the loss of her husband, Waneda was diagnosed with stage 3 breast cancer. For months on end, she lived in a fog. Nausea and the pain of her cancer treatments intermingled with waves of grief. During those dark hours, she believed life was essentially over.

Toward the end of her chemo treatments, Waneda had a vivid dream. In this dream, she was a young teenage girl again, back at her childhood home, lying naked in the front yard outside her bedroom window. As she lay still with arms outstretched, Waneda looked up into the sky and saw a bright light coming toward her. This light enveloped her, flooding her whole being with feelings of peace, warmth, and contentment.

Waneda awakened from the dream transformed. In describing this experience, Waneda explained that it was as if she had been reborn. After the dream, her deep grief was gone, and in its place was a new feeling of happiness. "I am fifteen. I am a happy fifteen," she told me.

I must admit that when Waneda described her dream and her feelings to me, I thought she was suffering from a form of denial. But as time went by, I began to see a new flourishing in Waneda's life. The cancer went into remission. A few months later, she quit her teaching job, sold her house, and moved to Zambia to work with children displaced by the AIDS virus.

Waneda's cancer was in remission for almost ten years. Thanks to the marvels of social media, I was in touch with her almost every day. I looked forward to her travel updates; her photos on social media contained images of beautiful children, many of whom were orphaned by AIDS. In every photo, Waneda is smiling broadly. As she entered her late sixties, Waneda seemed to have boundless energy. She enrolled in a PhD program and planned to focus her research on advocacy and children's rights.

Sadly, Waneda's cancer returned, and within a few months she passed away. I visited Waneda shortly before she died. She chided me that this book would not be finished before she passed to her reward. I reminded her that she was an inspiration for writing and promised her I would finish the book.

Waneda's dream revealed to her the second gift of menopause—namely, the gift of the authentic self. Her journey through menopause was marked with exceptional grief. Not only did she have to deal with the changes in her body, but her whole world was also turned upside down with the death of her husband and her breast cancer diagnosis. Waneda's dream helped her see that beneath the grief, sickness, and brokenness, the earlier, adventurous version of her self had not died. Instead, she was still very much alive and wanting to return.

Most women, as they enter midlife, do not have to deal with the major crises that were part of Waneda's life. Even so, menopause is a built-in crisis with enough transformational force to help us rediscover our deepest, most authentic selves.

As we age, we face the danger of becoming what Harriet Lerner describes as "de-selfed."[1] De-selfing happens when "too much of one's self (including one's thoughts, wants, beliefs, and ambitions) is negotiated . . . away."[2] By midlife, some women have negotiated away their wants, beliefs, and ambitions to the degree that they are no longer aware of their existence. They have become depleted selves.

Because de-selfing happens over the course of time, most women do not know they have become depleted selves. The storm of perimenopause is the jolt of awakening, lifting the veil from our eyes so we can see the ways the self has been given away. Marian Van Eyk McCain describes this awakening as the ending of "an automatic way of living where we left little room for reflection, no room for contemplation of the deeper self."[3]

If you take full advantage of the rough ride of perimenopause, allowing it to awaken you from an automatic way of living, you will find yourself eager for the gift of the authentic self. In order to receive this gift, you must be able to recognize the self.

Defining the Self

The self is the core part of our being. The self is the "I." It is our executive functioning apparatus, the part of us that makes us distinctive and separate from other people. Another word used to describe the self is *ego*. At birth, babies are in a symbiotic state with their mother. They aren't aware of where their body ends and the mother's body begins. Mother and child exist in a beautiful harmony of the "we."

Slowly, through the months, an infant's "I" begins to exert the power of separateness. Around the age of two, dramatic changes in the brain create a child intoxicated with the power of the "I." Spend any time around a two-year-old child and you will get a good dose of the ego. It is common to hear a two-year-old exclaim, "It's mine!" or "I do it myself." These phrases indicate the toddler has discovered the self and is attempting to develop independence.

As they grow, children must learn how to be in relationship with others while retaining a sense of individual identity. Adults who have a solid sense of self know how to give to others while at the same time not becoming depleted in the giving. Such people do not allow themselves to become absorbed by others. They are both the "not I"—people who give sacrificially to others—and the well-defined "I."

During puberty, the psyche of a young woman becomes primed for finding fulfillment in the relational web. At this time, the potent mix of hormonal changes and a cultural script that rewards compliant behavior puts the young woman in danger of having her ego repressed. There is a strong chance that she will emerge from puberty with a weakened and damaged sense of self. She may find it easy to exchange the "I" for the "not I."

Puberty is a perilous time for young women as they seek intimacy while at the same time attempting to retain a sense of self. They quickly learn that many young men seem to be threatened by women who have a strong ego. Young women learn to hide their intelligence or soften their voices in order not to threaten guys. They often feel they have to choose between having a strong sense of self and remaining single or submerging the self in exchange for marriage and children.

Our older daughter, Alethea, was a premed major in college. During this time, she would bring her friends over to the house for all-night study sessions. One young man was always over at our house. He seemed to have a very comfortable relationship with Alethea. Lest I get the wrong idea about their relationship, he told me, "Don't worry that I am after your daughter to date or to marry. She is as smart as I am, and I would never marry a girl who would not look up to me." At that moment, I thought to myself, *I am so grateful!*

As women, none of us are immune to the cultural influences that tell us it would be best not to have a strong ego. In the workplace as well as the home, women are encouraged to submerge the self to find approval. Through the years, we become good at reading social cues, knowing when to demur to those in authority, especially men. We become good at saying, "Oh, no problem. You go ahead and take the credit." When we reach midlife, we discover that we have become adept at giving away bits and pieces of our selves and that too many pieces have been given away. We are depleted selves.

We may be married or single, stay-at-home mothers or career women, but all of us, by the time we reach midlife, stand in need of the gift of the authentic self. Menopause is the time to re-self, to reclaim those bits and pieces of us so easily given away. This gift makes us more secure, grounded, and prepared for the journey into the second half of life.

How to Claim the Gift of the Authentic Self

I have identified five things you can do to nurture the self that is reborn during menopause: give yourself permission, provide the self the space and time it needs, connect with nature, set boundaries, and give yourself honor. These five actions will help you become a person who is able to navigate the give-and-take of relationships in a healthy, mature way.

Give Yourself Permission

A conservative Christian website recently posted information for women going through menopause. While the post had some good advice on healthy eating and hormone therapy, the author warned women, "Menopause is not an excuse for not serving." She went on to say, "Menopause may cause us to be very self-focused because we feel like the body snatchers have invaded. But, menopause is a time to look outside ourselves, to serve others as health allows."[4] In other words, keep on depleting your self because God honors self-sacrificing women.

The author of this blog post failed to understand how menopause is a divinely ordained pause to refocus on the self. It is common to confuse selfishness with developing a healthy sense of self. Because of this confusion, women miss the opportunities God gives them to become a transformed and mature person who is able to face the challenges of the second half of life.

A self-centered person is easy to recognize. She is all "I." She uses people to serve her own ends. Conversation revolves around her. She takes but rarely ever gives. A woman with a healthy awareness of the self gives to others while at the same time remaining aware of her own needs. She knows how to balance human relationships and remain intact. She knows how to balance her responses to demands on her time.

Awareness of the self is coming to a consciousness of one's core being, what McCain describes as a "sense of deepening, a sense of ever-increasing richness, like the maturing of fine wine."[5] My friend Waneda had a healthy sense of self. Whenever I was in her presence, I felt that I was with a person who was comfortable in her own skin. Her life energy was not being used in the quest for acceptance or approval. She radiated her own strength.

I am often with women quite unlike Waneda. They are the ones who never gave themselves permission to receive the gift of the authentic self. As a result, they are simply older versions of who they were in early adulthood. They are women who have aged, but they have failed to mature. They lack the depth and the richness of the postmenopausal life. They continue to expend their energy on keeping the seeming self going through reading the signals being sent by others and accommodating to those signals. In other words, they are not authentic.

Brené Brown defines authenticity as the "daily practice of letting go of who we think we're supposed to be and embracing who we are."[6] At first, the idea of letting go of who we think we are supposed to be can be quite frightening. How do we know that when we have let all that go there will be anything left? Maybe there is nothing there. Trust me. There is a great deal of your authentic self to be discovered. It is hidden underneath the layers of time.

Because authenticity is so frightening, we must have audacity— the shameless courage to become and stay real. Brown cautions, "Most of us have shame triggers around being perceived as self-indulgent or self-focused. We don't want our authenticity to be perceived as selfish or narcissistic."[7] Be aware of those shame triggers. They are what Brown describes as "a gauntlet of gremlins."[8] They are voices of judgment, criticism, and expectations. What they say can range from an off-handed comment about how you are no longer willing to stay late and clean up after the church potluck to harsh comments about your new "uppity attitude." In order to claim the gift of the authentic self, you must give yourself permission to challenge these voices and have the audacity to walk through this gauntlet.

During menopause, you have the choice. You can age, all the while taking a back seat in your relationships, or you can mature, embracing your authentic self that is seeking to return.

Provide Protected Space and Time

At perimenopause and beyond, you will discover that you crave more time alone. Don't ignore this craving or feel guilty about it.

The process of re-selfing is intense. It requires that we have not only the audacity to be authentic but also the audacity to move away from the crowd and be alone.

Many mothers dread the empty nest. I remember walking in the door of our house after dropping off our younger daughter at college and sensing a great emptiness. My daughter's absence was palpable; the rooms of our house seemed hollow. It took a while for me to adjust to this vast sense of emptiness. If this is a part of your experience, know that quietness provides opportunities for reflection and introspection necessary for developing the self. This newly found free time is part of the life cycle designed to help you focus on your inner life. It is designed to help you look deep inside yourself and find out who you really are.

For some women, perimenopause doesn't coincide with the empty nest. They go through the storm while raising teenagers. Things can get quite chaotic when our children's raging hormones meet our own. If this is your situation, it is important to carve out some protected time and space; otherwise, you will go through this season of life on autopilot. You will be in danger of missing the gift of self.

McCain calls this phase of the menopausal journey "the neutral zone."[9] The neutral zone is a space between times that allows us the luxury of stillness. In my journey through the neutral zone, I spent a great deal of time sitting in a large bay window in our family room. It was in this place that I felt safe to let the tears flow, express my anger, journal, and pray. I found the silent space to be a zone of comfort and a place of peace. In this space, no one demanded anything of me. I could simply be.

We grow accustomed to defining ourselves not only by our relationships but also by what we do. The neutral zone is a place to let go of the doing to focus on the inner world of being. It is a place for stripping down to our essential selves. Stripping down takes time—it is a process that cannot be rushed. Your inner self, long buried, will need time to come out of hiding. If you provide her with a safe and quiet place, she will gradually reveal herself.

The movement from the outer world into the inner world will require you to let go of images that no longer empower you. You will need to learn to develop the stronger power that is found only deep within. Developing this stronger power involves identifying and deconstructing those images that disempower you. During this time of my menopausal journey, I had to let go of images of perfection, control, performance, and achievement. In some ways, letting go of these things was not difficult. I had grown weary of living a life measured by the number of pages on my curriculum vitae. Academic rank, tenure, degrees, and titles had become measures of my self-worth. In the quest for these things, I was often plagued with anxiety regarding my value as a human being. By all appearances, I was a successful, high-achieving woman. But I was caught in a relentless quest for achievement.

During her life crisis, Lynne Hybels quit everything and entered the neutral zone. For months on end, she took up residence in an easy chair by a large window. "At first, I felt horribly guilty about these quiet unproductive moments. I tried to fight the exhaustion. I'd think, 'Okay, today I'll get busy again. I'll prove my worth again . . . ,' but I couldn't do it. I didn't have the energy."[10]

For many months, Hybels lived in her cocoon of quiet space. From her chair, she watched the summer leaves take on the colors of autumn. In the winter, she built fires in the fireplace, listened to music, sipped fragrant teas, and lingered over pages of art books. Sometimes she danced. At these times, Hybels felt like a little girl again—"not a nice girl seeking to please, but a playful child free to enjoy the simple pleasure of life."[11]

Although Hybels's transformation took place before menopause, her journey through the neutral zone offers a model for women who need to find their true selves. Hybels emerged from the neutral zone transformed from being a nice girl to being what she calls "a dangerous woman."[12] This dangerous woman now works as a humanitarian and peace activist.

The answer to the question "Who am I?" can be found only in the solitude of the neutral zone. As relational beings, we women find it difficult to carve out time in a quiet, solitary place, but that is exactly what we must do to claim our authentic selves. Work on giving yourself time to be alone in your own quiet place; claim this space as your cocoon, a place where new life can be born.

Connect with Nature

If we are not careful, our quiet places of solitude can become tombs where we bury ourselves instead of cocoons where new life is gestated. As we pass through the neutral zone, we must be careful not to withdraw into closed, claustrophobic space. Such space serves only to further our anxiety, and it may cause depression. For us to bring forth new life, we need both the protective space of our homes and the outer world of nature. These two spaces work together to restore the authentic self.

Connecting to the natural world is not easy. People today suffer from a malady Richard Louv calls "nature deficit disorder" (NDD).[13] NDD is characterized by diminished senses, attention difficulties, and higher rates of physical and emotional illnesses. NDD affects everyone, but I believe women, in particular, are prone to suffer from it. Men are encouraged to get out in nature—to fish, hunt, golf, and take part in other sports. Women, however, are encouraged to engage in indoor activities. Have you noticed how much of women's exercise, such as Zumba or yoga, takes place indoors?

Because many women have given in to this segregation of space, they often have dangerously low levels of vitamin D.

Vitamin D deficiency affects much more than the health of our bones and teeth. Low levels of vitamin D have been linked to obesity, diabetes, cardiovascular disease, autoimmune disease, and cancer.[14]

It is a strange irony that the wilds of nature are often the safest space for the emerging, fragile, authentic self. Nature is the ultimate restorative environment. It offers healing from our day-to-day anxieties as well as from our major life crises. Consider the words of Wendell Berry:

> When despair for the world grows in me
> and I wake in the night at the least sound
> in fear of what my life and my children's lives may be,
> I go and lie down where the wood drake
> rests in his beauty on the water, and the great heron
>   feeds.
> I come to the peace of wild things
> who do not tax their lives with forethought
> of grief. I come into the presence of still water.
> And I feel above me the day-blind stars
> waiting with their light. For a time
> I rest in the grace of the world, and am free.[15]

In nature, the self that was buried beneath layers of commitments, appointments, and relationships will feel free to emerge. The more time you spend in nature, the freer and more authentic you will become.

If you let her, nature will become your counselor, your friend, and your soul mate. During the heavy storm of perimenopause, she will provide you a safe place. She will listen to you, fill you with wonder, and soothe your pain. During my most difficult perimenopausal days, I discovered a nature preserve with trails that ramble beside a stream and through deep woods. Every day after work I would go there and walk for a couple of hours. This preserve became my separate peace—a buffer zone between the demands of work and home.

Nature has the amazing capacity to both expand the spirit and quiet the soul. In expanding your capacity for wonder and awe, nature moves you into a space beyond your own obsessive, negative thoughts. Women in perimenopause have a tendency toward obsessive thinking or what is sometimes called rumination. *Rumination* is defined as a pattern of often negative, inward-directed thinking and has been tied to an increased risk of depression. A recent study published in the *Proceedings of the National Academy of Sciences* indicated that people who took a ninety-minute nature walk showed a significant decrease in rumination.[16]

Nature can also quiet the soul. During the 1990s, the Japanese began studying how time spent in forests decreased blood pressure, elevated mood, and contributed to a person's overall well-being. The Japanese minister of agriculture, forest, and fisheries coined the term *Shinrin-Yoku*, which loosely translates as "forest bathing."[17] Forest bathing involves spending time in nature, exploring, breathing deeply, and meditating on the sights and sounds of nature. It is the process of soaking in nature.

Philip Bar, a physician specializing in integrative medicine at Duke University, is a forest-bathing advocate. In a 2017 interview with National Public Radio, Bar observed, "Forest bathing could be considered a form of medicine. And the benefit of nature can be accessed so simply."[18]

While exploring nature, I recommend you disconnect from your cell phone and forget about the tasks on your to-do list. This is the time of your life when something beautiful is emerging. Learn to walk at a slower pace. Explore new paths. Pay attention to the beauty of trees and the sounds of the birds. Become absorbed in the motion of a running stream as it cascades over rocks. Find a hidden tree and climb up into its tall branches. Let the restorative power of the tree embrace you. Learn to play again. Nature is out there, inviting you to move into her space, where you will discover a deep, ancient wisdom. Learn her ways and you will know yourself better.

Set Boundaries

Setting boundaries is perhaps the most important thing you can do to receive the gift of the authentic self. Boundaries are necessary. They are built into the cosmos. Our bodies have boundaries of skin that separate us from the world. The earth contains the boundaries of water, land, and sky. Countries have geographical boundaries. Cities set boundary markers. The land you live on is marked by boundaries.

Healthy people set boundaries, and they honor the boundaries of others. They know how to be in relationships without letting those relationships overwhelm them. They know the power of the word *no*.

People with good boundaries are more at peace with others and with themselves. They are more compassionate. Brené Brown points out how not having boundaries keeps us from developing the capacity for empathy. People without boundaries appear to be compassionate and caring, but they are often worn down and resentful from all the demands continually intruding on them. Brown writes about her 2007 breakdown, a time when she was forced to look at her lack of boundaries. "Before the breakdown," she confesses, "I was sweeter—judgmental, resentful, and angry on the inside—but sweeter on the outside." Now Brown sees herself as "genuinely more compassionate, less judgmental, and resentful, and way more serious about boundaries."[19]

Boundary-conscious people are more secure, more accepting of themselves and others. They are not always nice, but they are more frequently kind. "Nice" women do not have good boundaries. A lack of boundaries is what gives them the identity of "nice"!

Like Brown, you may discover that beneath your sweet outside resides an angry, judgmental woman. Menopause is a good time to exchange niceness and sweetness for kindness. This exchange involves learning to live with healthy boundaries. When you set boundaries, you construct protected space where you can grow and become healthy.

Be warned that the process of setting boundaries is hard work. You will have to learn how to use the word *no.* You will have to redefine relationships with other people. People who are accustomed to violating your time and space may react in confusion and anger to your boundaries. They will test the limits of your reserve to draw clear lines between their lives and your life. They will attempt to make you feel guilty for setting up border markers where there was once only open space.

Don't let the reactions of others deter you from setting healthy boundaries. The rewards of those boundaries will far outweigh the pain involved in creating them. With boundaries, you will discover that you are no longer living with the constant tyranny of the demands of others. You will find the freedom to have a more authentic, self-directed life.

SUSAN

As the oldest child in a dysfunctional family system, Susan grew up with a keen sense of responsibility. Her role in the family was that of the good girl and the fixer. As Susan's siblings grew into adolescence and adulthood, she assumed responsibility for their behavior, often apologizing to others or trying to make amends. As her mother aged, it was Susan who managed her care. Whenever anyone in the family needed help, they called Susan. Over the years, she bailed her siblings out of jail, fixed their bad debts, and lived her life on high alert for the next frantic call.

Moving to another state helped Susan establish some geographical boundaries, but modern technology made it possible for her family members to continue to invade her life with their demands. The demands from her siblings even enlarged to include their children. Susan became responsible for her aging mother, her siblings, and her nieces and nephews.

Crisis after crisis continued until finally, during the storm of perimenopause, Susan found herself unable to cope with the demands of her family. She began to see how her finances were strained, her marriage was suffering, and her own emotional well-being was at risk due to her lack of boundaries. Susan saw that she had three choices: continue as before until she collapsed, get help and learn how to set boundaries, or cut off her family altogether. While the latter seemed like a quick fix, she knew the healthier alternative was to fix herself and to learn how to set boundaries.

Susan entered therapy and began a journey of discovering how she had become so codependent with her family. She was forced to acknowledge how rescuing her family members fed her self-image as a caring daughter. Furthermore, she learned how this behavior kept her family in a cycle of codependence. While in therapy, she also discovered how her role of caregiver had been thrust upon her at an early age. She learned that it was not her responsibility to get other people to change or to clean up after their bad decisions. Susan faced the fact that she was responsible for her own actions and not the actions of others.

For Susan, setting boundaries with her family was a long and slow process. She had to learn how to love without letting others control her. She had to learn to say no. Most of all, she had to learn that the crises of others did not have to become her crises. It took years for

Susan to set definite boundaries and to keep those boundaries intact. At midlife, she found a new freedom of being. She no longer carried around a weight of guilt. No longer controlled by the demands of others, Susan found the joy and the freedom of a self-directed life. She faced her postmenopausal years with a newfound energy.

Setting boundaries is hard work. You may find that, like Susan, you need the assistance of a therapist to help you sort through all the voices of responsibility that have ruled your life. Don't feel guilty for seeking help. If Susan had not sought outside help, she would have continued in her unhealthy pattern of codependency.

Knowing where to set boundaries is difficult work. Like Susan, you may be tempted to build a wall of independence around yourself. This wall may solve the boundary problems, but it will isolate you from healthy interdependent relationships. Susan chose the route of interdependence and boundaries. A good therapist is a disinterested third party who can help you do the same.

In your journey toward self-discovery, learn to practice some of the following boundary-setting behaviors:

+ Become self-aware. Ask yourself, "What space do I need to be healthy and to maintain self-respect?"
+ When people place demands on your energy and time, take a moment to reflect on those demands. Are they made in expectation that you are responsible for fixing things?
+ Remember that your needs are valid. It is okay to have your time, your space, and your money.
+ Tell people when they are violating your boundaries. Let them know how their actions have invaded your personal space and time.

+ Stick with your boundaries. Do not allow yourself to be manipulated by guilt, and do not second-guess your decisions.

+ Respect the boundaries of others. You cannot expect other people to honor your boundaries if you do not respect their personal space and time.

Give Yourself Honor

In his conferences on Christian marriage, Emerson Eggerichs, author of the best-selling book *Love and Respect*, promotes the idea that the secret to a happy marriage is for women to honor their husbands and for men to love their wives. This bifurcated world where men need honor and women need love comes from Eggerichs's reading of biblical texts such as Ephesians 5:33: "Each one of you also must love his wife as he loves himself, and the wife must respect her husband" (NIV). "Paul is clearly saying," writes Eggerichs, "that wives need love and husbands need respect."[20]

In his Epistle to the Ephesians, Paul was not writing a description of the psychological nature of men and women. Rather, he was attempting to help Christians navigate the tensions between the ethics of Christ's kingdom and life in a pagan Roman culture. The gospel proclaimed a radical vision: "There is no longer Jew or Greek, there is no longer slave or free, there is no longer male or female; for all of you are one in Christ Jesus" (Gal. 3:28). But in the Roman world, men—the *paterfamilias*—ruled everyone in their household, including their wives, slaves, and children. Paul was attempting to modify this harsh reality by noting that wives should respect their husbands and men should love their wives. Likewise, slaves were to respect their masters, and their masters were to acknowledge that in Christ there was no free or slave person.

Eggerichs accepts the hierarchical model of the Roman household as normative instead of descriptive. He concludes that men have an innate need to be respected while women have an innate need to be loved. In order to give men what they need (respect), women should be quiet and respectful toward their husbands, even if they strongly disagree with them. Giving a man his due respect will garner his love. Women living in this outdated and bifurcated world between love and respect internalize the belief that respect is not their birthright. They believe that honor is the right of men. It is not to be returned to women, at least not on the same level. Men who believe that honor is their birthright work to reinforce the stereotype. As a consequence, far too many women have never felt honored. Sadly, they have never stopped to question why.

Honor is a human right. Everyone needs to be respected and honored for who they are. Every day I watch women, especially women who work for church organizations, go out of their way to honor men while at the same time never thinking to ask for honor in return. They settle for platitudes such as "You sure do know how to make things run smoothly around here. We need more ladies like you." These women diligently work behind the scenes, setting up for meetings and conferences, putting out materials, getting food together, all the while making sure that when the men walk through the doors, they find it easy to move into center stage and receive honor.

You may be a woman who believes honor is not your birthright. The gifts inside you may have never been sufficiently acknowledged, and you may believe that being in the shadows makes you more of a nice woman. You may believe that women who ask for honor and respect are pushy and aggressive. Yet deep down you crave honor.

Just as it is hard to set boundaries, it is hard to give yourself honor. Women are conditioned toward self-criticism. We are our own worst critics. Trying to measure up to a perfect ideal, we learn to be critical of our bodies, our actions, and even our thoughts. Consequently, low self-esteem is rampant among women of all ages.

Many women suffer from what Leonard Sax calls "anorexia of the soul."[21] This malady is a result of a false notion of perfectionism or a frantic search for an authentic sense of self that is never fulfilled. No matter how hard women try to be perfect, there are always elusive images of perfection just beyond our reach. The advertising industry is based on the assumption that life is a constant craving for more. Each season brings a new fashion or a new color that will make us more beautiful. The multibillion-dollar plastic surgery industry uses photoshopped images of older women who, using the marvels of Botox injections or surgery, manage to look thirty-five instead of fifty-five.

Women are never enough. We are never thin enough, caring enough, pretty enough, loving enough. The phrase "She wasn't enough for him" is often used to blame women for men's infidelity. Even in the Christian world, shaming is a tactic used to motivate women to work harder to be enough for men. I recently visited a blog that promotes how women can learn to be "a peaceful wife." It is the blogger's assumption that today's women, especially type A women—those who are driven to succeed—have to work extra hard in giving their husbands their due respect. The site is filled with blog posts telling women how they need to rein in their spirit, bite their tongue, and hold back their opinions, all for the sake of giving honor to their husbands and creating a peaceful home.[22] How is it that Christian women come to believe that being a type A woman is a deficit to marriage? Do we say the same thing about type A Christian men?

Attempting to measure up to every image of perfection will eventually split us women apart until we collapse upon ourselves.

Self-destructive behaviors, such as eating disorders and plastic surgery addiction, are on the rise as more women believe they cannot measure up to the ever-elusive images of perfection that saturate our society. The most dangerous move we can make is to dishonor ourselves. In doing so, we become filled with shame and self-loathing. Menopause is the time to take stock of self-loathing behaviors and to claim our right to honor. This is our time to turn attention to our selves with great kindness instead of harsh criticism.

During this time of your life, when the storm of perimenopause washes over you, you have the opportunity to discover the authentic self that got lost in the search to measure up to the standards of society. In the quiet wake of the storm, you can speak life and words of honor to your newly emerging and fragile self. You cannot wait for others to do so, especially if they have never spoken words of honor to you. It is up to you to honor yourself. If you can, pause for a few moments and say aloud, "I am a person worthy of honor!" Keep repeating this sentence until you believe it. If necessary, go outside and scream these words.

As you reflect on your inherent right to receive honor, analyze how you may have internalized outside criticism. Have other people's voices become so much a part of you that you do not know the difference between their voices and your own voice?

Separating yourself from the external critics is not easy, but it is possible. It is a process requiring you to make the important move from being an object to being a subject. An object is at the mercy of others. It has no inherent power. Things are done to objects. A subject, on the other hand, is self-directed. It acts instead of merely being acted upon.

Menopause provides the grand opportunity to become a subject. It gives you the space to reflect on how you may have allowed others to write a dishonoring script for your life. It gives you the opportunity to reflect on how, like an object, you allowed this script to define you.

Reflect on how you were taught to learn. Perhaps you were told to learn in silence, filling in the blanks of the information given to you. Perhaps you were told to respect the authority of teachers who had the "correct" information. As a result, you may have never learned to think critically, analyzing information for its strengths and weaknesses. You may have merely received information at face value. If you were taught to receive information without questioning, you are more likely to internalize outside messages about your own self.

JOANN

When Joann came to seminary, she worked hard to be liked by everyone. The word most used to describe her was *sweet*. Joann had a knack for flattering people in authority. All too often she would assume the stance of a too eager learner ready to give away her ideas to support the person speaking.

I enjoyed watching Joann make the journey from passive receiver to questioning student. In seminary classes, professors encouraged Joann to read and think critically. She was given permission to ask questions. During this time, she worked as my teaching assistant. I would often challenge her to express her own opinions and not merely the words of others.

During her second year in seminary, Joann was asked to attend a women's retreat. She did not want to go because, as she told me, she did not agree with all the teachings of the retreat leaders. But being "nice," Joann did not want to offend her relative who had agreed to sponsor her at the conference. She packed her bags and went to the retreat anyway.

A couple of days later, Joann called to inform me that she had been kicked out of the retreat. She described how, on arrival, each participant was given a workbook. As the speaker lectured, the women eagerly filled in the blanks, writing down the speaker's words verbatim. No one thought to question the speaker or to probe the material in search of deeper meaning. The retreat speaker never asked for questions. She merely encouraged the women to write down her words.

Joann resisted the expectation that she sit passively and fill in the blanks of her notebook. Instead, she practiced what she had learned in seminary—namely, asking probing questions, especially the *why* question. After the first morning session, the conference director took Joann aside and asked her not to be so disruptive. By midafternoon, Joann had been asked to leave the retreat. "You do not have a submissive spirit, Joann," said the director. "I encourage you to pray and ask God to give you more of a humble and learning heart."

When Joann shared this information with me, she was stinging from the rebuke. "Is there something wrong with me?" she asked. I encouraged Joann to notice how the conference was designed. The design revealed the mind-set that the women were receivers and not required to think for themselves. This design was not suitable for Joann, who, after attending seminary, had become an active, constructive learner. Perhaps Joann could have used more wisdom in her responses to the retreat leadership, but I was proud of her transformation.

Joann graduated from seminary and went on to become a denominational executive. In this role, she represented her tradition in international ecumenical venues. She now serves as a pastor. The journey from being a silent learner to being a critical thinker empowered Joann to believe in her own thoughts and to honor her own gifts. In other words, Joann had to become "a disruptive student" in order to become a good student!

The move to being a subject is a move toward honor and empowerment. This move is critical for your future well-being. It will make the difference between a life that is lived with purpose and one in which you merely parrot the ideas of others. You have the resources within you to make the move from object to subject. These resources are your own uniqueness, gifts, and abilities. There are also external resources, such as books by Brené Brown, designed to help you make the journey toward honoring your authentic self.

I have found the documentary *Miss Representation* helpful in revealing how media and advertising adversely affect women's self-images. The first time I watched *Miss Representation*, I was shocked at the ways women are portrayed in the media. I found myself asking, "Why didn't I notice this before?" This documentary helped me sort through the messages media sends to see what I had not been able to detect by myself. I often show this documentary to my students in classes on gender studies.

If you are uncomfortable with honoring your own self, begin with a few small steps. Start each day with words of affirmation. Begin the process of affirmation by speaking to yourself in the second person instead of the first person (e.g., "You are worthy and deserving of respect"). Speaking to yourself in the second person helps break the pattern of self-criticism. Whenever I criticize myself, I often use the phrase "I am so stupid." (Yes, I say these words to myself!) I am astonished at the difference this simple change in voice makes.

When speaking words of affirmation to yourself, avoid language that honors you for your roles or your actions. For instance, avoid saying things such as "You are a good wife" or "You are a great mother." Instead, speak words that reveal the qualities of who you are: "You are a person of great worth." "You are a woman of great valor and courage." "You are a wise woman." As you become more comfortable giving and receiving honor, you will find the power to switch to the first person: "I am a woman of integrity." "I am a woman filled with grace and love." As someone driven to perform, my favorite line of self-affirmation is "I am enough." I have it written on a yellow sticky note. From time to time, I pull it out and speak aloud the words. Sometimes I put the sticky note on my bathroom mirror where I can see it often.

A Word about Integration

Once you have discovered the "I" that went underground during early adulthood, don't think you have to banish the relational "not I." Instead, integrate the two. You can continue to be the nurturing mother, the loving wife, and the caring daughter. At the same time, you can be a woman who has clear boundaries. You can be a woman who thinks critically. You can be a woman who sees honor as her birthright.

Menopause is a good time to learn to reconcile the opposing forces governing your life. Sue Monk Kidd writes, "God calls us to the unifying and healing of our soul. God is *beyond* opposites. In God, everything is whole, is one. What's more, God made us for oneness, to know wholeness and harmony. God desires that we reconcile these opposing forces within us."[23]

Of all the gifts found in the journey of menopause, the gift of the authentic self is the most valuable. When you discover this gift, you have found a most precious commodity. You have found the person who will take you into the second half of life—a person with the courage, strength, and power needed to face a future that may look quite uncertain.

The gift of the authentic self is difficult to receive. Receiving it takes a great deal of energy and work, but it is worth the effort. Press into your pain from the gift of uncovering, channel the energy found in the gift of anger, and receive your one precious self who bursts forth. You will discover a person who is both admirable and strong. Only you have the power to bring her back to life. It is your voice that she knows best. She waits to hear you speak her name.

Personal Reflection Activities

1. What words would you use to describe your authentic self?
2. How have you experienced the process of de-selfing? What parts of your self have been given away over the years?
3. Describe the person you sense is being born at this time of your life. How is she different from the person you have been since adolescence? How is she the same?
4. Describe how you will give yourself protected time and space.
5. Describe how you plan to connect with nature. What places are available in your area for extended time in nature?
6. Revisit the section on boundary-setting behaviors and take time to reflect on each one.
7. Write a letter of honor to yourself. In this letter, speak words of affirmation to yourself.

Group Reflection Activities

1. As a group, discuss the ways women become de-selfed. Ask the following questions:

What parts of your self did you give away in order to find relational harmony?

What has been the cost of giving parts of your self away?

2. Discuss how menopausal re-selfing is different from selfishness.

3. Share experiences of the neutral zone. Reflect on them together.

4. Discuss the personal and the corporate cost of living without honor.

5. Review the section on boundary-setting behaviors. Name the behaviors that are the most challenging.

6. End the session with an honor ceremony. Write a sentence of honor for each of the women in the group. Form a circle. Take turns standing in the circle while the other members of the group read aloud their sentence of honor to the person in the middle.

FIVE

THE GIFT
OF EXPANDED
TIME

We cannot live the afternoon of life according to the program of
life's morning—for what was great in the morning will be little at
evening, and what in the morning was true will at evening be a lie.

—Carl Jung, *Modern Man in Search of a Soul*

MARY HALLAREN WAS THE FIRST WOMAN to achieve the rank of
colonel in the US Armed Forces. She also commanded the first
battalion of women sent to England during World War II. After
the war, Dwight Eisenhower asked Hallaren to oversee the up-
grade of the women's army auxiliary core (WAAC), an assign-
ment that would give women a permanent place in the military
establishment.

In an interview with Tom Brokaw for his book *The Greatest
Generation*, Hallaren recalled how her appointment was a hard
sell in the House of Representatives: "They felt the cost of integrating women into the service would be prohibitive because when
women reached menopause, they'd be worthless!"[1]

119

When the Hallaren hearings took place, great strides were being made in science and technology. However, in regard to views about women, advancement was slow. The view of menopause as "the death of the woman in the woman" was not confined to common folklore. It was also ingrained in modern medicine. During the mid-twentieth century, male physicians touted the need for hormone replacement therapy as a way of postponing the inevitable decline of women. Gynecologist Robert Wilson, whose research was funded by pharmaceutical companies, became a leading advocate for the use of hormone therapy to treat women suffering "the affliction" of menopause. In 1966, Wilson wrote an article for the *Los Angeles Times* lamenting how, at menopause, the very basis of a woman's selfhood "crumbles in ruin."[2] Menopause, noted Wilson, delivers "the end of womanhood." It causes a woman to be "suddenly desexed, a staggering catastrophe."[3]

Imagine living in a society where once women entered menopause, they were deemed disposable. Imagine the subtle and not-so-subtle messages conveying that older women were nothing but a desexed burden to society. Imagine the prevalence of coarse mother-in-law jokes in the media and from the pulpit. This world existed not too long ago. It was the world of my childhood.

Thankfully, beliefs regarding older women are changing. We are slowly getting the message that midlife, instead of being a time of decay, is actually a time for renewed energy and vitality. A record number of women are serving in the 116th Congress. Nearly a quarter of the voting members of the House of Representatives are women, the highest percentage in US history. A woman serves as Speaker of the House. Twenty-five women serve in the Senate. A seventy-year-old woman won the popular vote in the 2016 presidential election. Many of these women entered politics at midlife.

As you watch your body age, you may be tempted to believe the best years of your life are in the past. They are not. Menopause is not the bearer of death; it signals the arrival of renewed time. You no longer have the capacity to bear children, but the woman in you is not dead. You are entering a period of time that sociologist Margaret Mead described as being full of "post-menopausal zest."[4]

In Sue Monk Kidd's account of her own midlife crisis, she describes how, on the one hand, she was driven toward transformation. On the other hand, she was tempted to cling to the old, familiar ways of living. She writes, "We have within us a deep longing to grow and become a new creature, but we possess an equally strong compulsion to remain the same—to burrow down in our safe, secure places."[5]

The word *clinging* comes from the Anglo-Saxon word *clingan*, which means "shrink." "Clinging creates a shrinking within the soul, a shrinking of possibility and growth."[6] During the dramatic changes of menopause, it is often necessary to burrow for a while. Be careful, though. Burrowing easily becomes clinging, and clinging leads to shrinking.

In some segments of society, there continues to be the assumption that older women should cling to the script they were given in young adulthood. In these circles, older women are expected to channel their postmenopausal zest into the prescribed routines of their past. Menopause is not a time to cling to past images of womanhood. It is not a time to shrink. In fact, shrinking is the opposite of God's design for postmenopausal women. Women have a built-in alarm clock that begins to ring during menopause, signaling the expansion of time. Menopause expands time in two dimensions: cyclical and linear. The gift of cyclical time gives women the opportunity to become more in tune with the rhythms of life. The gift of linear time gives women the opportunity to get moving into the future. When a woman seizes the gift of expanded time, she is transformed into a mature, wise, and powerful woman. You can become that woman.

Cyclical Time

Think of a circle and you can imagine cyclical time. Cyclical time ebbs and flows, coming back around again and again. It is the time that marks the rhythms of day and night, the phases of the moon, and the seasons of the year.

Imagine a world in which we could not expect the sun to rise and set or a world in which we could not predict the seasons of the year. That world would be chaos. Cyclical time provides order. It provides stability, a steady ground on which we all live. Everyone benefits from cyclical time's regularity. Its predictability centers us. And its power soothes us.

Women, more so than men, are tuned in to cyclical time. We have been the guardians of its mysteries. Our bodies experience the rhythms of menstrual cycles, pregnancy, and birth. Just as does the moon, women's bodies wax and wane. The word *menstrual* comes from the Latin word *menses*, which means "moon's month." The cycle of the moon and most women's menstrual cycles are 29.5 days. Another name for menopause is "moon's pause."

"Time is a feminist issue," writes Jay Griffiths. "The male year is solar and counts months by the dozen. The female year is lunar and we have thirteen months."[7] Unlike today, time was once measured using both masculine and feminine categories. The days and months were measured by the solar calendar. The seasons and festivals were measured by the lunar.

In the old days, women were respected for their guardianship of cyclical time. Midwives were valued for their knowledge of the mysteries surrounding birth. People depended on women's knowledge of plants and herbs for healing. Older women were called on to read the signs of approaching death and to help guide the dying away from the land of the living. Well into the seventh century AD, feminine time was honored, but during the Middle Ages, things began to shift toward the masculine. Eventually, with the adoption of the Gregorian calendar in 1582, solar time was standardized and lunar time took a backseat.

The feminine disappeared not only from timekeeping but also from other areas. Male physicians gradually replaced female herbalists and midwives. Prejudice against older women increased. Those who continued to heal and deliver babies were labeled "rebellious hags" or "witches."

In 1486, the church published *The Hammer of Witches*, a guide for witch hunters. With this publication, the church wielded its power to help eradicate women who practiced the healing arts. The guide declared, "If a woman dares to cure without having studied, she is a witch and must die."[8] For over two centuries, women, and in particular older women, were the target of witch hunts. By the arrival of the seventeenth century, thousands of women had been put to death for the crime of witchcraft.

Despite these prejudices against women, people continued to live with a deep appreciation of cyclical time. They followed its signs—the phases of the moon and the alignment of the stars—for planting crops, pruning fruit trees, and castrating and butchering animals. These signs determined dates for marriage and the weaning of children.

In pockets of society, the signs continue to be valued. The *Old Farmer's Almanac*, first published in 1792, is the oldest continuously published periodical in North America. It serves as a guide to deciphering the signs. My husband consults the *Almanac* when planting crops, pruning trees, and sending cattle to be butchered. Farmers, midwives, heath care workers, and law enforcement officials are among those who continue the practice of reading the signs of cyclical time. It is no secret that emergency room personnel prepare for more patients during a full moon. Those who care for dementia patients are keenly aware of sundowners syndrome, a period right before sunset when confusion and agitation worsen.

In modern times, though, these signs are part of a superstitious past. People live devoid of any awareness of lunar time. They live without a lunar connection and don't pay attention to whether the moon is waxing or waning. They have no idea what a gibbous moon is. They don't know how the constellations are configured at any given time or how these constellations make their mark on a lunar calendar.

Few people acknowledge their deep connection to cyclical time. Rarely do people make an effort to greet the morning sunrise or stop to acknowledge a sunset. Who knows when bats come out of winter hibernation? Who watches for the arrival of migrating birds? Who can predict the arrival of a cold front?

We live in a society where the masculine world of productivity trumps the rhythms of the world of the feminine. As the saying goes, "Time is money." Artificial lighting creates an environment in which people don't have to worry about the darkness of night slowing down production. Environments built to control both lighting and temperature make sure production is not constrained by the seasons of the year.

In this 24/7 world, factories and stores are open around the clock. Even our homes rarely shut down! Cable TV provides around-the-clock entertainment and news. TVs are everywhere— kitchens, family rooms, bedrooms, and even bathrooms. The internet makes it possible for people to explore the unlimited storehouses of knowledge, connect with other people, and purchase goods at any moment of the day or night. Smartphones make it more difficult for people to shut down and recharge. It is common for people to carry their cell phones to bed with them. It seems that modern people, like factories and stores, are always accessible and open for business.

The existence of 24/7 time has led to changes in agricultural techniques. Industrial farmers can manipulate time. Day and night do not matter. Seasons of the year have no effect on the choices retailers can offer to consumers. Large-scale production of food, which utilizes a wide range of synthetic chemicals and artificially controlled environments, is part of this new world of farming. Thousands of animals, such as pigs and chickens, are raised in massive buildings where there is no night. These animals spend their entire lives disconnected from the natural world.

The endocrine system found in animals and humans is a built-in cyclical clock. It is a system consisting of glands that release hormones determining rate of growth and development. In today's industrial farms, growth hormones are injected into young livestock in order for them to gain fat faster or to produce more milk. When people consume milk or eat meat containing these growth hormones, their endocrine system is disrupted. Endocrine disrupting chemicals (EDCs) mimic natural hormones, but the way they bind to hormone receptors sometimes causes a more powerful response than does the original hormone. In other words, they can supercharge the endocrine system. These disrupters are found not only in the growth hormones injected into animals but also in the chemicals used to manufacture pesticides, plastics, flame-retardant clothing, and a host of other items. The human reproductive system is particularly sensitive to these chemicals. Many of the EDCs mimic estrogen. Estrogen-like chemicals found in plastic, food, and milk are causing early puberty in girls.[9]

Endocrine disrupters are also having an effect on the timing of menopause. A study conducted by the National Institutes of

Health in 2015 analyzed 31,575 women for exposure to endocrine disrupters. They found that women with high degrees of exposure to EDCs entered menopause two to four years earlier than those with less significant exposure.[10]

Living in a 24/7 world means we are always living on high alert, waiting for the next text message or the next demand on our time. This harried lifestyle creates more stress on our bodies. Stress causes higher levels of the hormone cortisol. High levels of cortisol cause more adverse symptoms during menopause, including intense hot flashes and depression.[11] Clearly, we are not created to be out of harmony with cyclical time.

How to Claim the Gift of Cyclical Time

Menopause is about letting go. You no longer have to worry about your monthly menstrual cycle. You no longer have to think about birth control. Menopause is also about claiming. The change provides a grace-filled opportunity to claim the gift of living in harmony with the deep rhythms of cyclical time. What follows are a few suggestions on how you can claim this gift.

Maintain Regularity Regarding Sleeping, Eating, Working, and Resting

During menopause, it is especially important to get to know your body and to learn how to work with its biorhythms. Every human body has its own unique rhythm of living in cyclical time. I am part of the 25 percent of the population who identify as morning people. I actually enjoy getting up early; my most productive time is during the morning hours, and it makes sense for me to reserve this period of the day for work that requires concentration. In the afternoon, I go into a slump. Taking a thirty-minute power nap after lunch gives me the energy boost I need for the afternoon. By 9:30 p.m., I am ready for bed. My husband, Jackie, is the opposite; he does his best work late at night and has a hard time focusing in the early morning.

During menopause, you will discover that you need more sleep. While you may be tempted to cling to your younger ways of forfeiting sleep in order to get things done, doing so is not wise. Insufficient sleep increases levels of corticosteroid and catecholamine—stress hormones that, when out of balance, wreak havoc on the immune system. Sleep helps with the maintenance of a healthy weight and restores both physical and mental energy.[12]

Practice Sabbath

Cyclical time is grounded in creation, not only in the regularity of day and night but also in Sabbath. In Genesis, Sabbath is the crown jewel of creation. It was the day when God rested and delighted in all that had been spoken into existence. Sabbath reminds us that creation is a gift. It calls for us to pause and acknowledge that we are not in control. We have our limits to making and doing.

In Jewish tradition, Sabbath (Shabbat) begins at sundown on Friday. At the beginning of the Sabbath meal, the mother of the house lights the Sabbath candle and invokes God's blessing. Sabbath is welcomed as the queen who descends from heaven to grace the world for twenty-four hours. She is the honored guest because her divine presence provides God's people with a joyful pause, a day of resistance against the tyranny of relentless work.

Years ago, I began practicing Sabbath. Every Saturday evening I would light the oil lamp on our dinner table. This simple action signaled that our family was entering a zone of special time. More recently, I have practiced shutting down all electronic devices from sundown on Saturday to Sunday evening. This time is my weekly neutral zone. Being away from the sounds of TV and radio and the distractions of social media gives me the opportunity to find a deeper level of peace where I can center my life and renew my strength for the week ahead. I usually take a long nap, not the weekday thirty-minute power nap, on Sunday afternoons.

You will find that as you take a day to rest—ceasing from work, shopping, and unnecessary activities—your body will begin to respond in positive ways. You will be less anxious. You will have more energy on the days following Sabbath. You will have more peace.

Pay Attention to Nature's Rhythms

The natural world not only keeps cyclical time but also celebrates it. "You make the dawn and the sunset shout for joy" (Ps. 65:8 NASB). Each morning creation throws a big party, complete with an array of brilliant colors streaking through the sky. Each evening the sky tunes up for another celebration. Each spring and fall, nature gets all decked out and throws a colorful banquet.

I fear we all will come to the end of our lives regretting that we did not pause to enjoy the times beauty shone through the crevices of creation. A few years ago, over a period of several hours, three massive tornados swept through our community, leaving a swath of death and destruction. Our property was sideswiped by the last and most deadly tornado. While our home was spared significant damage, all the pine trees in our front yard were either toppled or mangled. These trees had provided a shield between our house and the road. They hid our house so well that most people would drive by without realizing we were there. We liked being hidden from view.

With all the trees gone, we felt exposed. But Jackie and I soon realized that the hill our house sits on offers a front-row seat to magnificent sunsets. Being hidden behind the trees caused us to miss them. A couple of years after the tornado, we modified our house from a colonial with a front stoop to a farmhouse with a large wrap-around porch. Now sitting on the front porch and watching the sunset has become an evening ritual for my husband and me. We sometimes lament that we lived in our home for over fifteen years without noticing our grand view.

During your own "moon pause," slow down enough to admire the crocus pushing its way through the snow in early spring. Pause to listen to the first calls of the whip-poor-will on a summer night. By being grounded in the rhythms of the natural world, you will find you are more in harmony with creation. You will be less anxious and frazzled. You may even find yourself becoming, like your foremothers, a guardian of nature's secrets.

Avoid Farm Products Containing Endocrine Disrupting Chemicals

Living within the rhythms of cyclical time calls for us to become more aware of how we shop for food. A few years ago, buying milk or meat that did not contain growth hormones was expensive; organic produce was costly. Thankfully, today these products are within reach of the average consumer. Stores such as Trader Joe's and Aldi make special efforts to market hormone-free and organic products at low cost.

The Overextended Circle

During your menopausal journey, you will face the ever-present temptation to replicate the patterns and routines of an era that is ending. The children may have flown the nest, but you may desire to continue living as if nothing has changed. You may work

129

outside the home, but your work life is just another comfortable nest.

JANICE

You don't have to be in Janice's presence for very long before becoming aware of her nurturing skills. For decades, Janice supervised an early childhood education center. In this role, she showered love on inner-city children, many who did not have a stable home environment. In many ways, Janice was a mother to these children. She provided structure, affirmation, and much-needed affection.

Janice gave birth to two children of her own, a son and a daughter. Both children are now grown. As they graduated college, married, and entered their careers, Janice continued to nurture and support them in the same ways she did when they were young. She purchased their clothes. She bought their groceries. She assumed responsibility for their debts.

On the outside, Janice's children appear to be successful adults. They both have professional careers. However, a closer look reveals that Janice's children are not living as adults. Whenever they want a new car, instead of buying one they can afford, they ask Janice and her husband, John, to cosign a loan for a more expensive vehicle. Whenever an appliance breaks down, they call their mother for a replacement.

Janice works hard to keep her children in her nest. As grandchildren arrived, the nest enlarged to include them. To Janice, her grandchildren are her children. A few years ago, Janice took early retirement from her job as supervisor of a daycare center to provide free childcare for her grandchildren. This move put a strain on her finances; she and John had not saved for retirement.

Every Friday evening Janice's family goes out for dinner at a nice restaurant. It is assumed that Janice and John will pick up the tab. Whenever the extended family takes a vacation, Janice and John cover all the expenses.

To support his enlarging family and to compensate for Janice's loss of income, John began working two jobs, but at the age of seventy, he was diagnosed with cancer and had to let go of one of these jobs. Despite these changes, Janice is unable to evaluate her capacity to continue her role as primary caregiver of her extended family.

To maintain her mothering role, Janice is now overextending her credit cards. She and her husband are relying on a local food bank to help them get through each month. Month by month their debt level increases.

Janice is a woman who cannot let go of cyclical time. "Mother" is the identity from which she draws her self-worth. Janice's senior adult years are much like her life as a young mother, only now her energy level and her income are depleted.

Simone de Beauvoir, in her classic book *The Second Sex*, took note of women like Janice. She observed that after living only for their children, some women turn their full attention to their grandchildren, making no distinction between mothering and grandmothering. De Beauvoir pointed out that what appears to be self-sacrificing and loving behavior in older women is sometimes a bid for power. It is a bid for the only form of power they know—namely, mothering power. This bid for power is easily overlooked because it is cloaked within the framework of the caregiver and nurturer.[13]

Of course, not all parenting by grandparents is a bid for power. Sometimes grandparents serve as parents out of necessity. In a perfect world, our adult children would not die a premature death, they would not become addicted to drugs, a spouse would not abandon them. In a perfect world, grandchildren would not have to look to their grandparents to be their parents.

Ours is not a perfect world; sometimes our adult children are not capable of parenting, either physically or mentally, and when that happens, grandparents have to become parents. In 2019, more than 2.5 million grandparents were raising their grandchildren. Many of these children were victims of the opioid crisis in America. Grandparents are the unsung heroes of this crisis. As one grandmother remarked, "The bottom line of this whole thing is I didn't need another child; the child needed a mother."[14]

You may be one of the many women facing the challenges of raising grandchildren while going through the transition of menopause. It is hard to focus on the gifts of menopause while giving young children the attention they need. Your psyche and your body are preparing you for one way of being in the world while your responsibilities are the same as when you were younger. You may be ready to let go of the constraints of cyclical time, but your circumstances will not allow you to do so. Just as when you were younger, you have to rise early, fix lunches, and drive in the carpool.

If you are a woman raising grandchildren, keep in mind that things can't be the same as the first time around. Your body is not the same. Your psyche is not the same. For these reasons, it is important for you to seek outside help. You can't do it all. When you were younger, you may have done most of the childcare and housecleaning, but now you will need your spouse to be fully engaged in these things. Seek out support groups. Knowing that other people are going through what you are going through can help you feel you are not alone.

At this time in your life, you need to work on self-care, especially if you are raising young children. Self-care involves regular health checkups, exercise, and time away. When under stress, you may be tempted to let go of the rhythms of cyclical time, but these rhythms will help you stay centered. Regularity of sleep is important to keep your body in good shape. Keeping Sabbath is especially important. Shutting down what can be shut down will help restore you in both body and spirit.

At the same time, raising grandchildren can make you feel as if you are trapped in the routines of cyclical time. But time is moving forward. There are moments of pure joy. Live in those moments. Relish the love of family. Take delight in your grandchildren's laughter and pride in their accomplishments. As you think about your grandchildren's future, don't forget to plan for your own.

Linear Time

While menopause gives women space to live more fully in the natural rhythms of cyclical time, it also opens a door into another dimension of time—linear. Linear time moves forward. It has a past, present, and future. Think of a straight line and you will be able to envision linear time.

Linear time, as it moves from the past, through the present, and into the future, creates what we know as history. Men have been the lead actors in history. They have built the empires, fought the wars, discovered the new lands, and written the books. They are the ones who "go down in history" for their deeds. For these reasons, linear time is often referred to as male time.

It is likely you have heard the saying "Behind every successful man is a good woman." Men were able to live in linear time and make history because, in the background, women were tending to the duties of cyclical time. Women rose every morning and cooked breakfast. They had dinner ready in the evening. They birthed and nurtured children. They managed the cycles of cleaning the house and washing the clothes.

My grandmother had eleven children. She lived her entire life on a farm where her existence was framed largely within the drama of cyclical time. She knew the seasons for planting crops and butchering animals. My grandmother tended her flower garden with great care and was very proud of her poultry. She was a mother in tune with the earth and a nurturer of its life.

Although my grandmother's life was fulfilling, it was limited. She had little chance to participate in linear time. She didn't complete high school, and she never moved away from the farm or away from the lives of her children and grandchildren. My grandmother didn't run for political office, write a book, or make a scientific discovery. Other than adding lines to our family's genealogical chart and passing down her legacy in her descendants, my grandmother's life is not written in history books.

Unlike my grandmother, I was born in an era that gave me opportunities for living in linear time. During my young adult years, I had access to birth control, education, and a career. I was also able to choose the route of marriage and a family. This choice meant living in the tension between cyclical time and linear time.

We baby boomer women were free to step into linear time. We were allowed to do men's work—as long as it did not interfere with women's work! We were the generation of mothers who rose early, packed children's lunches, and drove them to childcare or school. Then, we worked all day and came home to make dinner, wash clothes, and clean the house. During the late 1970s and early 1980s, a TV commercial for the perfume Enjoli featured a woman touting, "I can put the wash on the line, feed the kids, get dressed, plant out the kisses, and get to work by five to nine. 'Cause I'm a woman!" The commercial ended with the words (spoken by a man), "Enjoli, the new eight-hour perfume for the twenty-four-hour woman."

Being a twenty-four-hour woman was exhausting. Looking back, I should have given myself permission to let go of many of the daily chores and trusted my husband to adequately handle them. He was more willing to assume household responsibilities than most men of his generation. But honestly, both of us were products of an era that continued to draw distinct lines between women's work and men's work.

You may be a woman who made the decision to focus on cyclical time, creating a gracious and warm space for your husband and children. You may be a woman who, like me, chose the route of living in both worlds. Either way, menopause is an opportunity to push the pause and reset buttons on time.

Menopause gives relief from some of the difficulties that come with juggling schedules of both cyclical time and linear time. You now have freedom to move more fully into linear time. If you chose the route of devoting yourself to the full-time care of loved ones, you will find that menopause gives you the opportunity to move beyond the nest. For all women, menopause offers the gift of linear time, complete with new callings and new adventures.

How to Claim the Gift of Linear Time

Linear time stretches out in front of you, calling you to move more fully into the future. Perhaps you are so accustomed to life as it has always been that you do not know how to step into that future. What follows are a few concrete suggestions on how to get moving.

Reexamine Your Routine

Cyclical time is determined time. It is the time that makes it possible to experience the deep rhythms of bleeding and participation in the renewal of life. Cyclical time makes it possible to have the security of a nine-to-five job and the assurance of a day-to-day routine. Sometimes this form of time slows us down.

At other times, it stops us in our tracks and traps us in its arms. Quite often these are lovely arms filled with warmth and great fulfillment. But these same arms can become restraints that keep us from moving forward into linear time.

Linear time is undetermined, open time. It leaves the future up to us. It calls us to accept responsibility over our own lives. It allows us to move from a life that has a predetermined script to one in which we write our own script. You may be accustomed to living out the script given to you by cyclical time. This script identified you as daughter, wife, mother, and grandmother. It may be a script of office worker or physician. At menopause, you can affirm this script while moving beyond it to a future that does not offer a prearranged plan. Now is the time to assess that script and write your own.

Take a good look at your life script and ask yourself the following questions: How am I living in time? Am I going through the motions, never stopping to think about the future? The answers to these questions are not found in any prearranged package. The answers are found in how you enter the story of your life: revisiting the past, clarifying the present, and envisioning the future.

Revisit the Past

The change is a time of assessing the choices we have made— our spouse, our career, our religion. The gift of uncovering is designed to help us look back at these choices with new clarity. Ask yourself these questions:

- What decisions did I make that I now regret?
- Are there things in my past that I need to resolve? If so, what can I do to resolve them?

+ How can I build on my past? What are the lessons I learned?
+ What things from the past do I need to let go of?

Clarify the Present

Linear time offers a landscape view of the present. At menopause, it is important to know who you are (self) but also where you are. Ask yourself some hard but necessary questions:

+ Am I in a good place? If not, how can I make my life better?
+ Am I satisfied with my job? If not, how can I find a job that brings fulfillment?
+ Am I happy to be a stay-at-home wife and mother? If not, how can I move into a more public space?

Envision the Future

In going through the motions of daily life, we often find it easy to push the autopilot button. The future becomes predetermined by the past. We don't have to take responsibility for its direction. Living in linear time calls for new levels of responsibility. With linear time, we cannot easily say that our role or our fate determines the future. In linear time, we determine our future.

As already mentioned, linear time is viewed as masculine. Men have honored and valued the power of linear time. In doing so, they have accepted responsibility for making history. With the cessation of menstruation and the empty nest, women gain the opportunity to become more masculine. Women can more fully enter the flow of history and assume responsibility for their destiny.

All human beings are a combination of masculine and feminine qualities. Some women are more masculine than others, but all women, including the most girly girls, have a masculine side. Within all women is a side that seeks to move forward and not just around. At menopause, women can honor their nurturing, nesting side while taking the risk to fly outside the nest.

Avoid Supermarket Time

Walk into most supermarkets and you will be greeted with the produce and flower section, a place where it is always midmorning in the merry month of May. Like produce and flowers, women are expected to look fresh and ripe and as if they are in the spring of life. We are expected to live in what Jay Griffiths calls "supermarket time."[15]

To move forward in linear time, you will have to let go of the illusion of living in the eternal bliss of supermarket time. It is not easy to let go of this illusion. While Western cultures have moved beyond the idea that older women are worthless, we have not moved beyond the expectation that older women continue to look young. These days it is fine to age, but we dare not look our age!

Only the strongest among us can resist the demands to look younger than our chronological age. Every month I am drawn to read a women's magazine published in the area where I live. There are always free copies on the stands in the foyer of the local YMCA. When a new edition arrives, I walk by the rack, look at the shiny cover, and tell myself, "You don't need to read this magazine. It only makes you feel bad." Every month I give in to the temptation to take a copy home. The magazine's beautifully designed cover and its large 17 x 14 size are just too much to resist. Opening and reading is like a journey through all the available medical procedures designed to make me look years younger:

breast augmentation, tummy tuck, Botox injections, permanent makeup, and artificial tanning.

Ads for these procedures usually include testimonies of women who have had the work done. My favorite ad features a woman surrounded by young children. The caption reads, "Can you believe she is a grandmother? Look thirty-five at fifty-five." Staring at the ad, I tell myself, "You could look younger. Work harder. Save the money and pay the price." (Of course, there is always a convenient payment plan.) Then reality hits me. This is the reality of my budget and the reality that no matter how much work I have done on my body, I will never again look thirty-five or even forty-five.

Because of the expectations placed on women to live in supermarket time, plastic surgery has become a multibillion-dollar industry. All around us are clinics, salons, spas, and treatment centers offering us the promise of a world where we are eternally thirty-five.

Take a look at an older woman who has undergone many plastic surgeries and injections. Like a mannequin, her face is frozen in time. She may not look her age, but she doesn't look any age. This woman continues the practice she developed years earlier—namely, the practice of creating a seeming self. Just as she did during her youth, she works hard to meet expectations of femininity, only now the price she pays for a flawless face, perky breasts, and a tight stomach is much higher.

The question for menopausal women is not "How can I avoid aging?" It is "How can I age with health, wisdom, and inner strength?" Supermarket time is no substitute for graceful aging. It may promise us a temporary fix for "the problem of aging," but it presents us with an even bigger problem—namely, the problem of denial. Denial creates inertia. It does little to help us move forward in linear time.

Each woman, as she ages, must make her own choices regarding health and beauty. As you make these decisions, know that not all plastic surgery and skin treatments are bad. If used properly, they can help you age with grace and beauty. Some women will need surgery for sagging eyelids or for sagging skin around the middle. Facial fillers are not necessarily bad. Just know that these things can become a substitute for authentic aging. As you age, avoid the trap of repeated surgeries or the idea that one more cosmetic procedure will guarantee eternal spring. Coming to terms with aging will help you enter the future with dignity and strength.

Strive for Authenticity in Look and Dress

We can no longer be a younger version of ourselves, but we can possess a quality of beauty that is remarkably handsome. Choosing to be handsome means that we work at developing a look that projects authenticity. There is nothing more beautiful than an authentic older woman. She radiates a confidence that beckons you to look beyond the lines on her face to see her inner light and wisdom.

Being authentic is not only about accepting frown lines and the inevitable pull of gravity but also about how we dress. Too many older women continue to dress in clothing that is designed for younger bodies. The resulting look is sometimes comical—think of sagging thighs pushed into tight leggings. Older women choose these younger styles because clothing options for postmenopausal women are often matronly dresses and drab suits.

There is some good news regarding women's dress: the growing trend, even among younger women, toward a style called menocore. Menocore combines normcore—unpretentious fashion—with the practical style of women going through menopause. Layers of linen, knee-length cardigans, and varied shades of taupe and indigo characterize menocore. This look is asymmetrical and sometimes boxy and gracefully combines femininity and aging. I have appreciated this style.

Younger women are also embracing the menocore look. In a recent article, a woman in her early forties described the look as "not only wearing comfortable clothes, but wearing clothes that signify comfort with yourself . . . a woman who has aged out of the male gaze without a backward glance, and she is totally at ease in her body. She exudes self-acceptance and self-actualization and all the other self-based issues we struggle with in our youth."[16]

Unfortunately, the menocore look can be expensive. But if you shop carefully, you can make it work on a budget. Not long ago, I stumbled onto an upscale used-clothing site where I found Eileen Fisher jackets (my favorite brand for the menocore look), normally retailing for four hundred dollars, listed for fifty. To make things better, the price is not fixed. You can offer a lower bid!

Stay Physically Fit

We older women can project a self-confident and handsome look, but doing so takes more than clothes and makeup. Now that I am in my mid-sixties, I have to pay careful attention to physical fitness. Type 2 diabetes runs in my family, as does heart disease. Being physically fit and having a healthy body weight are now important in preventing these diseases. To stay fit, I focus on both cardio exercises and muscle conditioning. Being healthy means that I cut down on refined sugars and carbohydrates. It means that I eat more lean protein and plenty of green vegetables.

Take the Risk

Moving forward in linear time requires a certain degree of risk. You will risk the criticism of others who want you to remain the same. You will risk failure. You will risk security. But in not taking the risks and living in the same mode as you did in the first half of life, you will certainly stagnate.

You cannot be the person you were in the first half of life. Too many things change, and the life patterns of your past will not be adequate for the future. In the words of Carl Jung, "What was great in the morning will be little at evening."[17]

Go ahead and grasp the gift of linear time. It stretches out before you as a wild and uncharted land. It is the land of your future, and it beckons to you.

Personal Reflection Activities

1. To what roles of the past are you tempted to cling?
2. Describe how you see yourself in five years and ten years.
3. List the changes you need to implement in order to live in harmony with cyclical time.

   How can you get out of the mad rush of 24/7?

   What needs to change in order to practice Sabbath?

   What about your rhythms of sleeping and waking?

   How can you pay closer attention to the rhythms of the natural world?

4. How might you be trapped in cyclical time? What changes do you need to make to move forward in linear time?
5. What about the future frightens you? How can you face these fears in order to move forward in linear time?

Group Reflection Activities

1. Discuss what it is like to live in premenopausal cyclical time: monthly periods, childbearing, daily childcare, and household chores.

2. Discuss the following questions:

   What parts of your earlier life are coming to an end?
   How can you move out of the constraints of cyclical time?
   How can you embrace the sacred rhythms of cyclical time?

3. Share any plans for the future. How does this future look different from the past?

4. Spend some time looking at life scripts.

   What was life like in the past?
   How are you living in time?
   Are you in a good place? If not, how can you make your life better?
   Looking into the future, how can you live with renewed purpose?
   How can you accept the responsibilities that come with linear time?

SIX

THE GIFT
OF SPIRITUAL
FREEDOM

Spiritual freedom only comes by following Christ outside the
gilded cage.

—Jackie David Johns, personal communication

Authentic God experience is always "too much." It consoles our
true self only after it has devastated our false self.

—Richard Rohr, *Falling Upward*

THE ARRIVAL OF MENOPAUSE gives women the opportunity to claim
the gift of expanded time. With this gift in hand, we can open the
door into another dimension of time: *kairos. Kairos* is an ancient
Greek term conveying "opportunity" or "season." In Christian
theology, *kairos* is used to symbolize "God's time" or "the fullness
of time."

Menopause is God's *kairos* for women. It is our season for an
in-breaking of the Spirit and greater spiritual freedom. Spiritual

freedom is the freedom of following Christ. It is the freedom of being led by the Spirit, the freedom to exercise the gifts the Spirit has given us.

The Good News Translation provides a vivid description of the Spirit's role in creation: "The earth was formless and desolate. The raging ocean that covered everything was engulfed in total darkness, and the Spirit of God was moving over the water" (Gen. 1:2). The storm of perimenopause has a spiritual dimension. During our time of deconstruction and chaos, fresh winds of the Spirit blow against the holding containers that have defined the parameters of our religious lives.

These Spirit winds seek to create new life and liberate us from the old patterns of living. In addition, they work to uncover the authentic spiritual self, a part of us that can easily be diminished by first-half-of-life tasks: marriage, raising children, establishing a career. During the first half of life, we may be active in church—attending Bible studies, volunteering, and participating in worship—but activity does not guarantee growth. In fact, being spiritually active is often a sure way of becoming numb to our deeper spiritual side. In all the doing, it is easy to overlook the being.

Like any other part of our lives, spirituality can run on autopilot, but after a while, inertia sets in. We begin to cling to well-worn clichés and spiritual platitudes. Remember, the old English word *clingan*, from which we derive the word *cling*, conveys shrinking. At midlife, most of us are in danger of spiritually diminishing. We find ourselves in need of a *kairos* moment. We stand in need of the gift of spiritual freedom.

Standing at the threshold of menopause, you may hear the Voice, "the one who unleashes a tune so spellbinding that we are compelled to follow, to stumble through shadowed corridors until we find the source of it."[1] Following this Voice means leaving the safe parameters of your religious landscape and venturing into uncharted terrain. If you choose to follow the Voice, your spiritual quest will be the most difficult, risky journey you will ever undertake.

The journey is difficult for two reasons. First, it is difficult because Western Christians are content to live with what Richard Rohr describes as a lower level of religious development, "one that is obsessively concerned with order, control, safety, . . . and certitude."[2] Western Christianity is disenchanted, hyperrational, and devoid of mystery. It runs smoothly—weekly worship services with liturgical options for every taste and programs for every age level. Our Christianity may be smooth, but it fails to create awe. We offer information, but there are few wise elders. We have a great deal of knowledge, but few of us experience the depths of mystery.

Second, the journey is difficult because Christian women live in a religious context that is hypermasculine. Contemporary Christianity eschews any reference to God as feminine. People have gone to great effort to defeminize biblical stories. Strong female biblical characters such as Deborah, Hulda, Priscilla, Phoebe, and Junia are ignored or distorted. Deborah, the judge, becomes an aberration, a fluke in God's will for women. Hulda, the prophet, is completely ignored. Priscilla, the teacher, becomes the woman standing behind her man, Aquila. Phoebe, the deacon, becomes the helpful servant. Junia, the apostle, is given a sex change and transformed into Junias, the male apostle.

Menopause is a time to let go of a religious life scripted by others. It is our time to write our own testimonies.

Women's Religious Seeming Self

During adolescence, girls discover that the price of relational harmony often entails submerging their authentic selves. Carol

Gilligan writes that because girls are often impeded from having powerful voices and disregarded in regard to their visions and dreams, they retreat into a metaphorical underground world. She describes this world as a place where girls keep their most precious thoughts and their own opinions.[3] On the outside, girls develop their seeming self. But on the inside, deep down in their psyches, there exists a different world from the one they project.

In her study of spirituality among adolescent girls, Patricia Davis discovered this underground world to be vastly different from the one on the outside. On the outside, girls appear to conform to religious codes, including purity codes. On the inside, girls are fascinated with the primal struggle between good and evil. Their underground caverns are teeming with issues such as sexual violation, poverty, violence, and injustice.

"Adults who tap into girls' fascination with the underground sides of life make a very good living," writes Davis.[4] The popularity of the *Vampire Diaries* television series, *The Twilight Saga*, and the *Harry Potter* books is indicative of girls' hunger for narratives that deal with danger, suffering, and the struggle between good and evil.

The newer *Star Wars* movies, with an adolescent girl, Rey, as the lead protagonist, allow girls to briefly bring their underground world to the surface. Rey's story embodies self-reliance in the face of abandonment and courage in the face of danger. Rey is chosen by the Force to inherit the mantle worn by a Jedi.

During my adolescence, there were no Reys in pop culture for girls to emulate. There were few narratives that tapped into our underground world. I was a huge fan of *Star Trek*, but looking back at the original series, I cringe at how women were portrayed. Female characters were sexualized, deceptive, and in need of Captain Kirk to rescue them. I was the teenage girl who longed to go "where no man had gone before." But to do so, I had to develop the lifelong skill of insertion.

Christian women learn to develop the skill of insertion early in life. We grow up singing:

> Father Abraham had many sons.
> Many sons had father Abraham.
> I am one of them, and so are you.
> So let's all praise the Lord.

Who paused to ask, "How might this song affect young girls?" No one. We all knew Father Abraham had sons. Not one daughter is named. It wasn't until Jesus healed the bent-over woman in the synagogue, recorded in Luke 13:10–17, that a woman is referred to as "a daughter of Abraham." Jesus spoke these words; they are subversively liberating.

Through years of inserting ourselves into stories and Scripture passages, we hone the skill of cultivating a religious seeming self. It is a self that smiles and sings along. It is a self that learns to bloom where it is planted, even in the shallow and rocky soil that fails to nourish the depth of our spiritual lives. In such soil, there is little hope for roots to grow deep enough to connect with our rich underground world. The religious seeming self is one that learns to adjust to what Carl Jung called "infantile surroundings."[5]

When the hidden caverns of women's spiritual lives are not explored, they become musty and closed off. Trauma, hard questions, tragic loss, and our own versions of *Nightmare on Elm Street* are hidden away down there. Other parts of our selves are also tucked away, such as dreams of being chosen by God to participate in God's wonderful project to heal a broken world. The good news is that the Holy Spirit dwells in those deep caverns. There she hovers over the hard questions and the pain. Her brooding wings fan the flickering flames of our deepest dreams, keeping them alive until we are ready to bring them to the surface.

Women do not venture into the deeper parts of their spiritual psyches because they believe that God expects them to develop a seeming self. They believe God requires them to diminish and that he delights when they make themselves small. Over the years, I have watched women exert a great deal of effort to repress those parts of their selves that were spiritually bold, assertive, and self-directed. They did so because they had been taught that God is pleased by such efforts.

Along with the religious seeming self, women learn to develop the religious seeming voice. Women are often keen to match expectations that they modulate their voices and lilt them upward. In many religious circles, women are especially attuned to expectations that their voices not convey any sense of spiritual authority. As one conservative pastor recently tweeted, "Women should be careful not to mimic the teaching authority of an elder."

BETH MOORE

Beth Moore is a woman of spiritual power. She oversees a large ministry, writes books and Bible studies, and speaks before thousands. Through the years, Moore had to learn how to navigate ministry in a religious tradition with tight restrictions on women: women cannot teach men, women cannot serve as senior pastors, women should submit to their husbands and to male leaders in the church.

In spite of these restrictions, through decades of hard work and Bible study, Moore managed to develop a thriving ministry. On the surface, she appeared to agree with the restrictions placed on her. But in October 2016, key Christian leaders, many for whom Moore had deep respect, voiced political support for a man who was caught on tape openly bragging about assaulting women. Moore began to see that behind the male façade of respecting and protecting women were attitudes that "smacked of misogyny." Moore had had enough. In May 2018, she posted "A Letter to My Brothers" on her website. She wrote, "As a woman leader in the conservative Evangelical world, I learned early to show constant pronounced deference . . . to male leaders and, when placed in situations to serve alongside them, to do so apologetically. I issued disclaimers ad nauseam. . . . I've been talked down to by male seminary students . . . [and] held my tongue when I wanted to say, 'Brother, I was getting up before dawn to pray and to pore over the Scriptures when you were still in your pull ups.'"[6] Moore managed to create free space where she could study and teach the Bible. But, as her words indicate, even she was not immune from the pressure to develop a nonthreatening religious seeming self and voice.

The restricted space of the seeming self contributes to a pervasive condition of arrested spiritual development. Far too many women enter midlife with the same form of spirituality they developed in adolescence—namely, one tied to the relational, pleasing self. Such women make good church members. They fit into the prescribed programs of "women's space." They teach children's church and sing in the choir or on the praise team. They participate in women's ministries and smooth out the rough edges of their faith communities.

All of us, both men and women, should be helpers, people willing to assist in the unsung business of living in Christian community. Some people have the gift of helps (1 Cor. 12:28). They prefer being in the background and are naturally gifted at making things run smoothly. The gift of helps is not gender specific. Some men have this gift. Some women have this gift. But there are women who have the gift of leadership. There are women endowed with the gifts of teaching and preaching. There are women who are called to be elders who share their wisdom with both men and women. Women whose gifts don't fit into the support-giving roles struggle to fit into the small, separated space where it is acceptable for their giftedness to be utilized.

Menopause presents the opportunity to take stock of your spiritual life. What are your deepest passions? What images do you have of yourself? What voice beckons to you? Does the spiritual place where you currently find yourself seem too small? Do you hunger for something deeper and more mysterious? Are you finding it hard to live within the spiritual space that characterized the first half of your life?

The Holding Containers of Women's Spirituality

Richard Rohr describes the first-half-of-life spirituality as a time of "holding containers." Holding containers are "the faith given to us." They are constructed out of traditions, group symbols, family loyalties, and civil and church laws. Holding containers provide a sense of "goodness, value and special importance of your country, ethnicity and religion."[7]

Holding containers are good for us, especially when we are young. They provide security, identity, and tradition. Holding containers draw the lines, setting secure boundaries of rules and doctrine and ideology. Without these lines, people are prone to a haphazard life on a constant quest for identity.

There comes a time, however, when the spirituality of morning is wrong for the afternoon. Earlier in life, we may have tolerated or found refuge in easy answers, platitudes, slogans, and prescribed feminine roles. The complexities of later life compel us to search for a spirituality of the mysterious, the deep, and the wonderful. We hunger for amazement and a sense that we have a place in the grand drama between good and evil.

For us to grow, to experience the things for which we hunger, our first-half-of-life holding containers have to give way. The winds of perimenopause are designed to facilitate their breaking apart, and when they do, we are able to move out of the shallows and launch into the realm of greater spiritual freedom. This spiritual journey is not for the faint of heart. It takes a courageous soul to go where you may be required to forsake your spiritual homeland and chart a new course toward undiscovered worlds.

It is easier for men to venture beyond institutional boundaries and explore what is out there. They can do so without having their sense of masculinity threatened. Going out may even earn them the envied labels "pioneers" and "visionary leaders." The rulekeepers of their institutions may question nonconventional men, but at the same time, they will allow, or even praise, their movement beyond the boundaries of their own tribe.

BILLY AND RUTH GRAHAM

Billy Graham is an example of someone who dared to explore the world beyond his religious holding containers. On the one hand, Graham remained grounded in his conservative Baptist faith. On the other hand, he moved beyond the boundaries of his own tribe. Over the decades spanning his life, Graham traveled the world and met with world leaders. During the Cold War, he ventured into the forbidden spaces of Communist China and the Soviet Union. While Graham experienced criticism for his unorthodox ministry, he was known—for the most part—as "a prophet with honor," even in and among his own people.[8]

Just as Billy Graham is an example of a man who dared to go beyond the holding containers of his early life, Graham's wife, Ruth, is an example of a woman who accepted the restraints of her religion's feminine holding containers. While Billy was away, Ruth stayed at home and raised the children. Moreover, Ruth questioned women who chose paths outside their roles as wives and mothers. In an article she wrote for *Christianity Today*, Ruth offered her opinion of a woman's place: "I think if you study you will find that the finest cooks in the world are men (probably called chefs); the finest couturiers, by and large, are men; the greatest politicians are men; most of our greatest writers are men; most of our greatest athletes are men. You name it, men are superior in all but two areas: women make the best wives and women make the best mothers."[9]

Ruth Graham penned these words to counter the growing feminist movement of the late 1960s and early 1970s. It was a time when women were daring to move outside of traditional roles. Women were developing a public voice. Some women were even asking to be ordained as religious leaders. In the midst of these cultural shifts, Ruth's softly modulated voice contained a biting rebuke of women who were tempted to leave conservative evangelical feminine holding containers.

The Holding Container of Patriarchy

A few years ago, Jackie and I visited a local church on Mother's Day. I expected the exoneration of motherhood. Most Mother's Day services are beautiful—honoring older mothers as well as younger ones. I thought I might even come home with a flower or a scented candle. Never in my wildest imagination could I have dreamed what actually happened.

The theme of the Mother's Day service was "What Every Woman Wants for Mother's Day: A Man to Lead Her." Men led the service. A men's choir sang "manly" songs such as "Onward, Christian Soldiers." At some point during the service, the pastor asked all the men and boys to stand in a pledge "to lead women well." My husband and an older man in a wheelchair were the only men left sitting.

After the pledging ceremony, the pastor announced that a young couple had brought their newborn baby girl to church. He went into the congregation and gently lifted her so that everyone could get a good look at the church's newest addition. Even though I was stunned by the previous events—the male choir, the men's pledge—I was most grieved by this event. Here was a baby girl, fresh out of the womb, and already her spiritual fate was determined.

Jackie and I were happy to escape from this church service. On the way home, we talked about how women had sat passively during the Mother's Day program. Not one woman spoke publicly during the service. In many churches, Mother's Day is the only time women are allowed behind the pulpit or given a public voice other than in singing. But at this church, Mother's Day was co-opted in order to reinforce their silence—all in the name of gifting the women!

Mother's Day at this church in Cleveland, Tennessee, serves as exhibit A of a culture of patriarchy. Patriarchy may be broadly defined as a general system in which women are subordinated to men.[10] The English word *patriarch* is derived from the Greek word *patriarches*, which literally means "the rule of the father." Patriarchy is as old as humankind. It is found in all the world's major religions. In Judaism, Christianity, and Islam, conservative theologians tout patriarchy as God's design.

There are variations in the degrees of patriarchy. There is the hardcore form that considers women the property of men. Proponents of this brand of patriarchy believe that women's ontological status is inferior to that of men. In other words, women are not the same kind of human beings as men. In previous centuries, this belief about women was common. The ancient Greeks viewed women as inherently defective, closer to animals than to men. All cultures of the ancient Near East understood women to be morally, intellectually, and physically inferior to men. Women were the property of men. It was in this world that the Bible was written.

One can still find places where hardcore patriarchy flourishes. Several Middle Eastern countries have rigid rules and laws governing the behavior of women. Women live under the supervision of male guardians. They cannot travel, go to the hospital, or make a major purchase without the explicit permission of their guardian.

Benevolent patriarchy is common in modern Christianity. It teaches that women are full human beings, made in the image of God. But proponents of benevolent patriarchy call for distinctions in roles for men and women. Sometimes this form of patriarchy is called complementarianism.

Proponents of benevolent patriarchy assert that male rule was established before the fall of Adam and Eve. They teach that sin distorts God's beautiful design of men leading and women joyfully submitting. Benevolent patriarchs make little distinction between the context of the Bible—namely, ancient patriarchal culture—and God's intentions for humanity. They read Paul's discussion of Roman household codes in the New Testament as a reflection of God's design and not as Paul's attempt to navigate the freedom of the gospel in a world where men—the *paterfamilias*—ruled. In their estimation, God's beautiful design for women draws clear lines between men's and women's authority and spheres of influence. Things are clear—patriarchy is God's doing.

Whether in its hardcore form or its more benevolent form, patriarchy is undergirded by the belief that women are designed by God to be supervised by men. The image of "being under" dominates patriarchy.

+ Women are designed to be under the leadership of men.
+ Women are safer under the protection of men.
+ Women best serve God under the guidance of men.

In both its hardcore and its benevolent form, patriarchy is also undergirded by the belief that women should be silent.

+ Women should limit the range and tone of their voices.
+ There are certain places where women are not to speak.
+ Women should not challenge men, especially in public.
+ Women should modulate their voices so as not to convey authority.
+ God expects women to limit their authoritative voice to the spheres of women and children.
+ A woman's authoritative voice is never to be used when addressing men.

The Holding Container of the Good Woman

In a patriarchal world, the best way a woman can survive is by being good. The good woman is an older, more mature version of the nice girl. The nice girl is someone who works at maintaining her seeming self. She is good at picking up on social cues and responding to outside expectations. At a certain age, the nice girl turns into the good woman. The good woman has an air of maturity about her, but not enough to threaten men. As an updated version of the nice girl, the good woman continues to find her self-identity in male affirmation.

I have worked in the context of benevolent patriarchy my entire adult life. Let me tell you something. Benevolent patriarchs love good women, women whom they can count on to act in a certain way:

+ good women who work behind the scenes to make things happen
+ good women who stand behind their men

+ good women who don't ask too many questions, especially in regard to inequity
+ good women who are hardworking, God-fearing, and dispensable
+ good women who are the smiling assistants
+ good women who work to make themselves thin, unseen, and unheard
+ good women who believe their value comes from the men they serve

Within patriarchal cultures, the image of the good woman is clothed with spiritual significance. God's design for women is that they are first and foremost good. God is portrayed as the great benevolent male who approves of

+ good women who work behind the scenes to make things happen
+ good women who stand behind their men
+ good women who don't ask too many questions, especially in regard to inequity . . .

I could go on, but I'm sure you get the picture.

If you live in a context where people teach benevolent patriarchy as God's design, you may be frightened to step outside its boundaries. Deep down you may believe that in doing so you will incur the displeasure, even the wrath, of God. I would recommend you read the book *Malestrom: Manhood Swept into the Currents of a Changing World* by Carolyn Custis James.[11] Custis James does an excellent job of tracing the history of patriarchy and showing how it has been a destructive force for both men and women.

The Quest of Midlife Spirituality

At menopause, women stand at a crossroads. Will we simply age into the role of the good woman? Or will we seize the window of opportunity offered by menopause's clearing winds and claim the gift of spiritual freedom?

If we choose the road toward spiritual freedom, we will move from a place where we learned to color in the lines to a place where the lines are fluid. We will discover that the faith we developed earlier in life can no longer adequately portray God's wonderful mysteries. Stories, symbols, and ideas once taken for granted will seem insufficient in the new world.

Sometimes dramatic events such as the death of a child, abuse, or a divorce create enough impetus to journey away from the safety of one's spiritual home. Events such as these have a way of revealing how the spaces created by religious holding containers are not large enough for deep pain or complex questions. They may also reveal the spaces of those religious holding containers to be toxic.

Today, more women are daring to question the gatekeepers of their spiritual holding containers. They are mustering the courage to step outside the gates. The presidential election of 2016 and the ensuing #MeToo and #ChurchToo movements served as catalysts for women to question their religious leaders. Over the last few months, I have watched as middle-aged women have begun to wrestle with the deal they made in early adulthood: "We played by the rules. We have stayed within the boundaries of God's design for women. Meanwhile, men are promoting a double standard for themselves."

The #MeToo and #ChurchToo movements have thrown open the doors on women's repressed anger. Stories of abuse flood social media. The stories reveal how women are now seeing their religious holding containers as unsafe spaces. The religious gate-keepers of these holding containers are scrambling for explanations. It is painful to watch.

Recent sexual abuse scandals have generated enough disillusionment and anger to create an exodus from conservative evangelical churches. While the exodus is well documented regarding millennials, it is easy to miss the growing number of older women who have taken leave of the religious traditions in which they once found meaning and fulfillment.

Other older women have chosen to stay within their traditions, but they do so stripped of their earlier naivete. Both those who have departed and those who have stayed are in search of a spirituality that offers a deeper, more humanizing way of being in the world.

These days I find myself in conversation with women who, having left the secure dwellings of their first-half-of-life holding containers, find themselves spiritually homeless. A few months ago, I spoke at a conference largely attended by younger ex-evangelicals. Hidden within the over two thousand attendees were numerous older women. Several of these women found their way to me for extended conversation. Their stories are heartbreaking.

Brenda, a woman who grew up Southern Baptist and who was ordained as a pastor in a Southern Baptist church, became spiritually homeless during the conservative takeover of the Southern Baptist Convention. Although it has been nearly twenty years since Brenda's banishment from pastoral ministry, she has not yet found a spiritual home. "I am Baptist to the core," said Brenda. "I did not leave my denomination. They left me."

Brenda is one of the many older women who have left the known world of the past and have not been able to find another home. Opening the gates of their first-half-of-life spiritual holding containers, women such as Brenda have dared to leave behind the comforts of home and set out on a journey to a new land. They find themselves in a valley of doubt and fear. They don't know how to express the world they are seeking. They only know it is there, behind the mysterious Voice calling to them.

You may be a woman disillusioned with the first-half-of-life holding containers. You may have one foot out the door. You may be well on your journey toward that mysterious Voice. Or you may feel disoriented, as if you have just landed in a foreign country where the rules of your earlier life have no meaning. You don't even understand the language of this new space. Everything within you screams, "Turn around and go home! It may be a tight space, but at least you know that world!"

Trying to ignore these thoughts, you continue walking outside the gates leading from baggage claim. We all bring baggage from the holding containers. Here you are surrounded by a cacophony of voices offering to be your guide to your new spiritual destination. Some of these voices seem trustworthy. Others? Not so much. Who can you trust?

The Christian world is full of self-proclaimed spiritual guides for women. Upon closer inspection, you notice that many spiritual guides are a lot younger than you expected them to be. As much as you value their voices, you find yourself asking, "Where are the older women, the ones whose faces mirror my own?"

I am one of those older women. You can find me standing outside baggage claim. I am holding up a sign that reads, "The gift of spiritual freedom." I offer myself as a guide in your quest. I want to help you find a new and better home.

I am on my own spiritual quest, but I am far enough along to give you some solid advice. In short, I am asking you to travel with me on this journey toward greater spiritual freedom. It is my hope that along the way you will develop an enlarged vision of God, embrace an enlarged vision of yourself, and learn to embrace paradox.

Before we begin this journey, I need to remind you of something: holding containers have guardians and rule keepers. When a questing woman steps out on her spiritual journey, she has to leave behind the voices of the guardians calling out, "Don't go beyond these limits!" "Women are not allowed over there!" "What do you think you are doing?" And there is my favorite question: "Who do you think you are?"

A woman who dares to go beyond the voices will find herself on a road less traveled. But she is not alone. Along this journey she will find traveling companions, others who are seeking a more mysterious and deep space. She may discover the gift of wise elders who are willing to serve as her guide. If she is sincere in her quest, she will eventually discover the presence, the companionship, of the Holy Spirit.

Shortly before his death, Jesus met with his disciples and instructed them about life after he was gone. This discourse is found in John 14–17. It is sometimes referred to as the Paraclete sayings or the final discourse. Jesus warned his disciples that their first-half-of-life spiritual holding containers were going to break apart. A great shattering was coming—his death. Jesus told his disciples not to fear what was coming. A new world was on the horizon. It was a large, spacious place filled with many rooms. The world of God's eternal presence was drawing near, and Jesus longed to share this sacred place with his disciples.

In the meantime, Jesus wanted his disciples to know that he would not leave them alone. He was sending them "another Comforter," the Holy Spirit (John 14:16). The Spirit would be the disciples' traveling companion, leading them into all truth. The guardians of the old order would lash out with accusations. But the disciples were not to worry, for the Spirit would give them the right words to say.

As you journey outward toward the beautiful world of sacred presence, God will not leave you orphaned. He has sent the Holy Spirit as your traveling companion. Over the years, in my own spiritual quest, I have found the Holy Spirit to be a steady, abiding presence. Sometimes the Spirit bursts into my life with dreams, words of prophecy, and visions. More frequently, the Spirit is an enveloping and sustaining presence. Sometimes I feel her presence brooding over me. When I am enveloped in grief, she is there— God grieving with me.

A few years ago, I had a dream that changed my life. I was riding a bus through a large city. The bus was crowded with many passengers, but as it made frequent stops, people would get off. Eventually, I was alone on the bus and traveling outside the city. Gazing out the window, I could see no houses. There were no people around. At some point, the bus stopped. The driver turned to me and said, "It is time to get off." As soon as I stepped off the bus, it disappeared. I stood and looked around. As far as my eyes could see, there were no signs of civilization. Feeling overwhelmed with fear, I cried, "I am alone! Totally alone!"

As soon as those words left my mouth, the skies lit up in glorious colors. The fields came alive with color. Music filled the air, and I heard these words: "If my father and mother forsake me, the Lord will take me up." I began to dance. It was not the beauty that caused me to dance, nor was it the music. As promised, I was being taken up, swept into a divine dance. Since that dream, I have lost loved ones. I have suffered stinging criticism from the guardians of the spiritual holding containers. At times, I have lost my way. But I have never felt orphaned. The Lord has taken me up.

The questing woman has to leave behind her need for institutional security. Knowing that the spiritual holding containers offer no permanent home, she follows Jesus by going outside the gates. The way of Jesus takes her into a place where she bears shame and criticism. In the end, however, the gift of spiritual freedom is worth all the hardship. Once you find this gifted space—your lasting city—you will never want to return to the safe world of holding containers. The new wine Jesus has in store for your second half of life cannot be held in the old first-half-of-life wine containers.

How to Claim the Gift of Spiritual Freedom

You may want to leave the constraints of the first-half-of-life spiritual holding containers, but you aren't sure how to begin. What follows are suggestions for taking the first tentative steps toward claiming the gift of spiritual freedom: enlarge your vision of God, enlarge your vision of yourself, and embrace nondualistic thinking.

Enlarge Your Vision of God

To find your new spiritual home, you will need to enlarge your vision of God. The image of God mediated by the gatekeepers of your first half of life is not adequate for the mysterious realm of second-half-of-life spirituality. God is deeper, wider, more wondrous than you can imagine. There are no holding containers adequate for knowing God.

Western Christianity has a distorted vision of God. Our God is hypermasculine, and theologians work hard to eradicate any feminization of Christianity. God is not male or female—God is Spirit (John 4:24). Yes, God is most often imaged as Father, and Jesus was a man. But as a Roman Catholic sister so poignantly stated, "Surely God is more than two men and a bird."[12] While God is not a man or a woman, God has both feminine and masculine attributes. It is helpful for us women to name the feminine attributes of God; in doing so, we can more easily see ourselves as humans made in the image of God.

In my husband's study of feminine images of God in the Bible, he drew the following conclusions:

> The Scriptures contain many references to God that are explicitly feminine in character. They all flow out of the creation account where we are told humanity, male and female, is created in the image of God (Genesis 1:26–27). God speaks of Himself as having a womb (Job 38:29) and of giving birth (Deuteronomy 32:18). He compares Himself to a nursing mother (Isaiah 49:15). He cries out like a woman in the labor pains of birth (Isaiah 42:14). He repeatedly describes Himself in the role of a midwife at the birth of a child (Psalm 71:6, 22:9–10, Isaiah 46:3–4, 66:9–10). He fulfills the role of a mother or nanny nourishing and teaching Israel like a young child (Hosea 11:1–4). He comforts like a mother comforts her child (Psalm 131:1–2, Isaiah 66:13). He is as the mother eagle who cares for and teaches her young (Deuteronomy 32:11–12) and He protects His own like a mother bear protects her cubs (Hosea 13:8). Jesus speaks of Himself as a mother hen who would gather her young to herself (Matthew 23:37, Luke 13:34). These feminine images of God do not make Him female any more than the masculine images make Him male. All of them serve to communicate to us that our God is a personal God to whom we can relate. How sterile would our knowledge of God be if we did not know Him both as father and mother, masculine and feminine?[13]

Feminine images of the Holy Spirit. Two Hebrew words used in the Old Testament are translated "spirit": *ruach* and *neshamah*. Both words are feminine in the Hebrew language. In the New Testament, the Greek word for the Spirit, *pneuma*, is neuter, neither masculine nor feminine. Thus, the prevailing grammatical references to the Spirit in the Bible are as a "she" and certainly not as a "he."[14]

As the doctrine of the Trinity developed, early Christians made a point of referencing the Holy Spirit as a person and not as an "it." God eternally exists as three persons: Father, Son, and Holy Spirit. In the early centuries up to about AD 400, the personhood of the Holy Spirit was predominantly thought of in feminine images. Syriac Christianity, in particular, was rich with feminine imagery of the Holy Spirit. Sebastian Brock writes, "In the two surviving manuscripts of the Old Syriac Gospels the Holy Spirit is invariably treated as feminine."[15]

In the West, masculine images of the Holy Spirit gradually replaced feminine ones. As Latin became the dominant language of Christianity, the feminine images of the Spirit were lost. The Latin word for spirit, *spiritus*, is masculine. The shift to masculine images for the Holy Spirit also involved a reaction against heretical teaching, such as the belief that the Spirit of God was the Mother and that Jesus was the product of the sexual union of God the Father and the Spirit.[16]

In my own life, feminine images of the Holy Spirit have been both comforting and empowering. The Holy Spirit is God's all-embracing, creating, brooding, transforming, convicting, and comforting presence. During my perimenopausal storm, the Holy Spirit drew near. She became God's radically imminent presence in my life. She kept me under her wings; she brooded over my brokenness, stirring up life. She comforted me during the long nights of pain, tears, and anger.

On the other end of the menopausal journey, the Holy Spirit liberated me from the tight holding containers of women's spirituality. She empowered me to find my voice and to speak my truth. Such is the work of the Spirit as feminine—holding on to us and freeing us, comforting us and empowering us. She keeps us under her wings long enough for us to heal and then at the right time releases us and launches us out into the world.

The mystery of the relational God. Another way of imaging God is to look at God as "Being in Communion—the 'We.'"[17] God is a trinity—three persons in one. Writes Elizabeth Johnson, "Speaking about the Trinity God is not a solitary God but a communion in love marked by overflowing life."[18]

God's relational life is sometimes referred to as *perichoresis*—a term implying co-inherence of the three divine persons, the encircling of each around the other. The life of God is oneness and unity, a beautiful, eternal dance of the three persons of the Trinity.

In God's overflowing life, it is the Holy Spirit who reaches out and pulls humanity into the divine dance. The Spirit brings humanity to God and God to humanity. We abide in the life of God, and God's life becomes our home. Here we experience the nearness of God, what theologians call God's immanence.

Remember the gift of puberty—the relational self? Did you know that when you received this gift, becoming a woman who loved and gave of herself to others, you were imaging God? You were imaging what Ann Bedford Ulanov describes as "the female element of being," a constitutional part of God's very being. In fact, this nurturing element of being is the sacred foundation of life. She writes, "God's love, like a mother's, goes into us and establishes our being. . . . God's love establishes being as a gift. Love precedes being, creates being, and passes being on through the female element."[19]

Consider the words of Clement of Alexandria, who lived during the second and third centuries AD: "For what further need has God of the mysteries of love? And then thou shalt look into the bosom of the Father, whom God the only-begotten Son alone hath declared. And God Himself is love; and out of love to us became feminine. In His ineffable essence He is Father; in His compassion to us He became Mother. The Father by loving became feminine: and the great proof of this is He whom He begot of Himself; and the fruit brought forth by love is love."[20]

A man and a woman who live in a long-term relationship have the opportunity to facilitate and admire the "not I" in each other. Sometimes the mother soothes the crying child. At other times, the father rushes in to comfort her. My mother gave birth to me. She nursed me in an era when doing so was not popular. My father, who had been a medic in World War II, was the chief soother of the family. It was he who held me during the rough days and nights of chicken pox, measles, and mumps. During those times, he would sing to us what we called his silly songs. The sound of my father's voice lingers in my psyche. His soothing touch remains in my sense memory.

The mystery of the separateness in God. At midlife, you may discover how your relational self has left little room for the authentic self. You may realize how the "I" got lost in the "we." At this time in life, you may be drawn to re-self and claim the parts of you that were too easily given away. That part of you emerging as the "I" is also the image of God in you.

God is the relational "we," but God is also the "I." God's triune life is not one of enmeshment. It is one of boundaries, respect, and individual personhood. Father, Son, and Holy Spirit are three distinct persons of the Trinity.

The distinctive "I" found in God and in humanity may be described as "the male element of being." Writes Ulanov, "We may identify with the other, but we do not become the other. An I and a You exist, and we do things to and with each other and know about each other."[21] The "I" of God emphasizes transcendence over immanence. It is that aspect of God that is distinct from the world. It is the part of God's life that honors the boundaries of the other members of the Trinity. The male element of being is God honoring the free will of humanity. It is the foundation for honoring the individuality of every man and woman and child.

During midlife, you may discover how your individual self became absorbed into the lives of others. Such a life is not healthy. It lacks boundaries. It fails to acknowledge your ideas and your unique gifts. Re-selfing rights the imbalanced life. It gives you a needed dose of the male element of being. Just as both women and men carry the female element of being, we all carry the male element of being.

Just as in the life of God, where both the female and male elements of being comingle, humanity is a beautiful harmony of both elements. Menopause is the time for women to become more like God—and claim the "I" without letting go of the "we." For us women to be fully human, we must live as integrated and whole beings.

Enlarge Your Vision of Yourself

Many women struggle with developing a healthy self-image because they struggle to have a healthy image of God. The understanding we have of God is closely tied to our self-understanding. For instance, men often see God as "someone like me." From childhood men are exposed to male images of God in art and in language. The most common theme in women's vision of God is "someone not like me." Women who have grown up in a culture of patriarchy find it hard to imagine they are made in the image of God. They say, "Of course, all people, both men and women, are made in God's image," but they don't really believe it. Deep down most Christian women are convinced they are not fully made in the image of God, at least not as fully as men.

Just as we women work to insert ourselves into Christian songs and biblical stories, we work to insert ourselves into the image of God. We hear, "God created man in his image," and deep inside we shout, "Me too!" The truth is we don't have to insert ourselves. From the very beginning, we were there: "So God created humankind in his image, in the image of God he created them; male and female he created them" (Gen. 1:27).

Heirs with Christ Jesus. In the time when the New Testament was written, it was unthinkable for women to be heirs of an estate. In a Roman household, the estate went to the sons, with the eldest son having preference. Wives and daughters were socially and economically weak. In fact, they were considered a part of the estate! If there was no son, a Roman man would adopt a male, usually someone in his extended family, and make him the heir.

Jesus gave us the gift of eternal life; he also gave us a new household—where we can live out the gift of eternal life. The apostle Paul went to great lengths to contrast the household of God to the Roman household. God's household is quite different. It is a household in which Jesus, as elder brother, shares with all of God's children the fullness of inheritance: "For all who are led by the Spirit of God are children of God. For you did not receive a spirit of slavery to fall back into fear, but you have received a spirit of adoption. When we cry, 'Abba! Father!' it is that very Spirit bearing witness with our spirit that we are children of God, and if children, then heirs, heirs of God and joint heirs with Christ—if, in fact, we suffer with him so that we may also be glorified with him" (Rom. 8:14–17).

Peter reinforces the same message of women as joint heirs: "Show consideration for your wives in your life together, paying honor to the woman as the weaker sex, since they too are also heirs of the gracious gift of life—so that nothing may hinder your prayers" (1 Pet. 3:7). In Greek, the word *asthenel* is used for

170

"weaker." It is a term for someone without social or political power. Prisoners were *asthenei*, slaves were *asthenei*, and women were *asthenei*. Peter acknowledges that women have a lower/weaker social status, but he admonishes husbands to live out the new order of creation, one in which women are also heirs of the gift of life. I can only imagine how hard it must have been for men to wrap their minds around the idea that their wives were joint heirs with them. I can only imagine how hard it was for women to grasp the truth of their new status.

A royal priesthood. In terms of life in the new order of creation, Peter makes another radical claim. He writes, "But you are a chosen race, a royal priesthood, a holy nation, God's own people, in order that you may proclaim the mighty acts of him who called you out of darkness into his marvelous light" (1 Pet. 2:9). Just as Jesus made a way for a new kind of household, he also made a way for a new order of priests. In the Old Testament, only men from the tribe of Levi served as priests. Women were not permitted into the priesthood. However, in the new order of creation, all those in Christ's large family—both women and men—are not only heirs with Christ but also part of a royal priesthood.

I can only imagine how hard it was for women of the New Testament era to grasp the truth that they were part of a priesthood of believers. Unfortunately, it is sometimes hard for women living in the present era to see themselves as part of a royal priesthood. I often hear, "The husband is the priest of the home." The belief that men serve as priests—mediators with Christ—for their wives has a great deal of traction within evangelical Christian circles. However, it is another example of theology without any scriptural foundation. No biblical text references a man as the priest of his household. Christian women, whether they are single or married, have the same priestly status as men. We do not need a male mediator between God and us. There is only one high priest—Jesus Christ. There is only one mediator between humanity and God—Jesus Christ.

To move into your time of spiritual freedom, you will need to claim your identity as both an heir of the new creation and a member of Christ's royal priesthood. These two identities will provide the security you need to travel beyond spiritual holding containers. The apostle Paul wrote, "There is no longer Jew or Greek, there is no longer slave or free, there is no longer male and female; for all of you are one in Christ Jesus. And if you belong to Christ, then you are Abraham's offspring, heirs according to the promise" (Gal. 3:28–29).

Embrace Nondualistic Thinking

The world of women's spiritual holding containers thrives on the use of dualistic thinking. The capacity for dualistic thinking develops around the age of twelve. It is part of what psychologist Jean Piaget described as "formal operational thinking."[22] Formal operational thinking enables a young person to think beyond the concrete and the literal. At its first stage, the level of dualistic thinking, a young person frames the world in binary categories. They learn to compare and contrast things. They enjoy sorting through ideas and making judgments about things.

The capacity for dualistic thinking is empowering and a bit intoxicating. Middle school kids suddenly know everything. They can easily become obsessed with judging and comparing. They compare their parents to everyone else's parents. Because of these capacities to compare and contrast, kids at this age make great debate team members. Theirs is a world of black-and-white, "those like us" and "those not like us."

Dualistic thinking helps people make rules. It is the type of thinking helpful for determining right from wrong, good from evil. Most institutions operate within the realm of dualistic thinking. They reward people for playing by the rules and playing on "their team." The world needs dualistic thinking. Without it, people would live in chaos.

Nondualistic thinking is the second level of formal operational thought. It builds on the foundation of dualistic thinking but goes beyond it into the realm of possible convergences. Dualistic thinking splits things apart; nondualistic thinking puts things together. Nondualistic thinking appreciates this statement attributed to Niels Bohr: "The opposite of a profound truth is often another profound truth." The same statement completely frustrates a dualistic thinker.

Nondualistic thinking is required for studies in higher mathematics, physics, and philosophy. Higher education, in its best forms, cultivates such thinking. Throughout history, women were denied access to higher education; in being denied higher education, most women failed to develop nondualistic thinking. As a matter of fact, for most of human history, higher-level thinking in women was viewed as an aberration of true femininity. The German philosopher Immanuel Kant wrote, "Laborious learning or painful pondering, even if a woman should greatly succeed in it, destroy the merits that are proper to her sex. . . . They weaken her charms with which she exercises her great power over the other sex. . . . A woman with a head full of Greek . . . might as well have a beard."[23]

Even today, it is more difficult for females to develop nondualistic thinking than males. Girls are rewarded for staying within systems. The terrible choice offered to young women, to be either feminine or adult, reinforces dualistic thinking. Likewise, for young women to become "spiritually feminine," they have to hone the skills of dualistic thinking. In many religious traditions, nondualistic thinking is the forbidden fruit for women.

Over the years, it has grieved me to teach women with obvious high levels of intelligence and extremely low capacities for non-dualistic thinking. I have to work extra hard in encouraging them to think outside the box and to research new ideas. At some point, most of these women, both old and young, begin to resist the move to nondualistic thinking. One middle-aged woman would sign up for classes, attend a few weeks, and then drop them. In investigating the reasons for her behavior, I discovered that at some point her professors would disagree with the theology of her minister father. She was driven to be the good daughter, and holding an opinion different from that of her father was unthinkable.

The number of female college students continues to rise. So much so, that for the first time in history more women are enrolled in college than men. In 2017 the ratio of female to male college students was 44 percent to 37 percent.[24] Women are becoming adept at nondualistic thinking. There are cultural ramifications associated with this shift. Young women are no longer content with prepackaged answers. They see themselves as thinking subjects who act upon the world. As a result, more women are questioning their spiritual holding containers. With the rise of internet-based social media platforms and blogs, more women are finding the freedom to express their ideas and challenge their religious traditions. This shift has taken male religious leaders by surprise, many of whom are not accustomed to being questioned by women. Nondualistic thinking thrives on paradox. Paradox may be defined as the creative joining of opposites. Martin Luther King Jr. wrote, "Life at its best is a creative synthesis of opposites in fruitful harmony."[25] Spiritually mature and free people live in the beautiful tension of paradox: suffering and joy, dying and living.

Reading Paul's letters, one cannot help but see how he learned to embrace such paradox. Because of his ability to live betwixt and between, he was able to elder a young church. He was able to steer believers through the tensions of law and grace and to embrace those they once held in suspicion.

You may be a woman who did not receive permission to think nondualistically. You may find it hard to appreciate paradox. Deep down you may believe that letting go of the black-and-white categories and prepackaged answers is equivalent to having a critical spirit. I encourage you to let go of the need to hold on to prepackaged answers and to seek a deeper way.

Second-half-of-life spirituality is filled with paradox: knowing and not knowing, searching and finding, community and solitude, restraint and freedom. When a woman learns to embrace the betwixt and between of paradoxes, she is on her way toward becoming a wise, spiritual elder.

Personal Reflection Activities

1. What words would you use to describe your spiritual life?
2. Describe how you see yourself living in your first-half-of-life spiritual holding containers.

How have these holding containers provided safety and identity?

Who are the guardians of your first-half-of-life spiritual holding containers?

What images of women are conveyed in these holding containers?

In what ways are these holding containers becoming too small?

What fears do you have about moving beyond the holding containers?

3. How has your life been affected by patriarchy? Do you see the need to move beyond it?

4. Describe how you see yourself as made in the image of God.

5. What are the personal costs of claiming the gift of spiritual freedom?

6. Have you understood yourself as the good woman? How has this vision of yourself affected your spiritual life?

7. What needs to change in your life in order for you to develop a greater capacity for nondualistic thinking? How is this form of thinking important in your life at the present time?

8. Envision yourself as part of a royal priesthood. What would it mean for you to live in this vision?

Group Reflection Activities

1. Spend some time reflecting on the first-half-of-life spiritual holding containers.

2. How have these holding containers been helpful in finding identity and providing security?

3. How have you outgrown the first-half-of-life spiritual holding containers?

4. In what ways have they become toxic?

5. Discuss the expectations placed on women to stay within the first-half-of-life spiritual holding containers.

   Why is it threatening to others for women to go beyond these containers?

> How is it difficult for women to go beyond these containers?
>
> Who are the guardians of your containers?

6. Name the ways women are made in the image of God.
7. Discuss how God has both masculine and feminine modes of being.
8. Write a description of what it would be like to live in the gift of spiritual freedom. Open the floor to anyone who would like to share her vision of spiritual freedom.
9. End the session by praying for one another.

SEVEN

THE GIFT
OF VISION

The place God calls you to is the place where your deep gladness
and the world's deep hunger meet.

—Frederick Buechner, *Wishful Thinking*

AFTER HER DRAMATIC DREAM in which she discovered her earlier
self, my friend Waneda moved into a new phase of life, one that
took her on an amazing journey. She was a tireless advocate for
children's rights and never stopped looking for ways to use her
gifts to help others. Waneda was a woman of remarkable intelligence and bravery; moreover, she was a woman of vision.

Caroline is another woman of vision. After retiring from teaching school, she was awakened to the plight of those who struggle
every day to live on wages that are so low they must choose between buying food and paying their utility bills. She began volunteering every day at her local food bank, and the people who
regularly visit the pantry find her to be a calming presence and a
person with whom they can talk. They know she will not judge
them for needing food assistance. She is their friend.

Caroline not only serves the poor in the food bank but also is active in a local group of people who are advocating for an increase in the minimum wage toward a "living wage." Caroline often finds herself in situations where people strongly disagree with her stance on the living wage, but she stands her ground. "A few years ago, I never would have had the courage to become politically active. But now, well, I just don't care so much what other people think of me. I care more about how I can live with myself."

Vision is not something for a few people like Waneda and Caroline. It is for ordinary women who believe in an extraordinary God.[1] Women entering the second half of life are uniquely poised to receive this gift. Having received the gift of expanded time, you are ready to move forward with a purpose. Having left the constraints of the first-half-of-life spiritual holding containers, you are ready to set your sails toward a new, more fruitful land.

Menopause is a time when women can discover a beautiful and holy calling that will guide them in the journey of the second half of life. This time of life offers the possibility of living for a cause that is larger and grander than our own self-fulfillment. Dale Hanson Bourke points out that the vision we acquire for the second half of life is "a holy calling rather than what other people may believe you should be doing."[2] Discovering one's holy calling is not always easy. Women who have lived out prescribed roles may find it difficult to see beyond the roles and to embrace a vision. Acquiring a vision means we have to let go of living out other people's visions and find our own. Sometimes menopausal women need to go on a vision quest.

Menopause as a Vision Quest

The practice of a vision quest originated in Native American groups as a rite of passage between childhood and adulthood. It is a compressed time in which youth spend a designated period alone in the wilderness, seeking spiritual guidance and identity. Going through a vision quest is difficult. It stretches one mentally, physically, and spiritually. A vision quest opens the possibility of finding one's identity and calling. It marks a person for life and gives birth to a new name.

Vision quests are a unique blending of the inner and outer worlds. The inner world is engaged through fasting, meditation, and solitude. Sometimes hallucinogenic agents such as the peyote weed are used. The outer world is the world of nature, the world of the elders, and the spiritual realm. The Lakota Sioux word for vision quest is *Hembleciya*, which means "crying for a dream." The authentic self that was uncovered during the storm of perimenopause is fragile, but she is not passive. She is crying for a dream, for a life not characterized by the prescribed roles of years past. Her cry may be masked by the business of life, but menopause is a built-in time when she can stop, purify herself of baggage from the past, and turn her attention to the heart's cry.

When I entered the terrain of my journey toward menopause, I did not know that my body would be taking me through what amounted to my own personal vision quest. My journey toward menopause was characterized by some of the same markers that often characterize Native American vision quests. During perimenopause, I had no sweat lodge, but there were plenty of night sweats. My body was purifying itself in preparation for a new life. I did not fast or take hallucinogenic agents, but due to hormonal changes, my mind was filled with invasive and vivid images, memories, and thoughts.

Like those who participate in vision quests, I spent a great deal of time alone in nature. I spent a great deal of time in solitude at home during which I wrapped myself in quietness. Like a butterfly pupa in its cocoon, I was in a stage in which things within me were dying and other things were being born. What I did not have for my menopausal vision quest was a community of elders or spiritual directors. Women in Western society have been relegated to silence regarding menopause. For that reason, we have no spiritual guides to help us through the menopausal journey. We are left to go it alone through a significant developmental period of our lives.

What could be a rich, rewarding, and challenging experience often becomes a time of confusion, muddled thinking, and embarrassment. Nature did not design it to be this way. Imagine what our lives would be like if women could go through the menopausal rite of passage surrounded by elders and spiritual guides. Frankly, such things are too dangerous in societies that disempower women. It is not easy to change a society that is devoid of women elders or vision guides; we can't replicate what a community of elders would give as we walk into our vision quest. We are left to find guidance in friends and in books. This book is designed to serve as a spiritual and developmental guide for you as you undertake your vision quest.

In this chapter, I will be asking you to go inward, to look at, in the words of Frederick Buechner, the place of your "deep gladness."[3] I will be asking you to look outward, over the horizon of your busy life, to see the world's needs that may be beckoning to you. In this space, where the inward and the outward meet, you will find your vision and calling for the second half of life.

Spending time at a retreat center or a remote place where you can be alone will help facilitate your vision quest. If you can take the time to get away, carry nothing with you that can distract you from the quest. It is important to unplug from social media, TV, radio, and other outside distractions. If you know you will have a difficult time disconnecting from the frenzied world of technology, find a place that does not offer these distractions. These places do exist! The best things to carry on your vision quest are your Bible and a notebook.

How to Claim the Gift of Vision

Look Inward: Find Your Passion

A vision is the core of life that guides all our actions. It judges all our tasks, commitments, and appointments. A vision strips us down to the essentials, to the things that really matter. It frees us to let go of many distractions. Moreover, it unburdens us from the guilt we often carry as we begin to live out of our own expectations and not the expectations of others.

Discovering your vision involves simplifying, subtracting, and cleaning out. Seeking a vision is not about adding another exciting thing to your bucket list. A vision is not another item on your to-do list. A vision is who you are to become. Discovering a vision is not the same thing as an adrenaline high. It is not a frenetic activity that quickly burns out. Actually, finding the sweet spot of your passion slows you down, causing you to be more settled and focused.

Writes Parker Palmer, "We are disabused of original giftedness in the first half of our lives. Then—if we are awake, aware, and able to admit our loss—we spend the second half trying to recover and reclaim the gift we once possessed."[4] With these words, Palmer aptly describes our menopausal journey: we awaken and become aware, we admit the loss of our authentic selves, and we move toward the recovery and the reclamation of the gifts that are rightfully ours and ours alone. We discover our vocations, our holy callings in life.

If you have set boundaries around your fragile self and if you have given her protected time and space, there is the possibility that she will begin to speak to you, guiding you toward your deep gladness. She will help you take the first tentative steps toward discovering your vision.

Your authentic self may not be accustomed to being heard. If so, her first words will emerge as a whisper. Listen to this voice, no matter how small or tentative. Give your authentic self permission to speak about herself. Many women have learned to speak in the voices of others to the degree that they may not know the sound of their own voices.

Your authentic self will begin to speak by telling you what no longer matters to her. When I began listening to my inner self, the first whispers that emerged were, "I am so very, very tired." With the help of a good therapist, I learned to listen to this voice. My therapist helped me make the painful discovery that I did a great deal to please others; this way of living had left me exhausted.

I discovered that for decades I had lived according to what may be called the tyranny of others. I had allowed other people to define my activities, my schedule, and my identity. After many years of this behavior, I did not know the difference between my inner passion and the outer expectations placed on me. They had become one and the same.

My therapist helped me see that this pleasing behavior was my default or automatic mode of being. I am the eldest child in a dysfunctional family. Growing up, I became adept at reading what was expected of me. I became a high achiever but never felt that I quite measured up to others. I spent the first half of my life grasping for one more approval rating. I wish I had a dime for every time I heard, "I don't know how you do it all." Striving to do it all was a way toward self-validation. However, the validation never came because there was always one more demand, one more request for my attention.

Pleasing everyone is hard work. It required me to live on high alert to the expectations of others. At any moment, I was ready to commit myself to a multitude of tasks: speaking engagements, writing assignments, serving on committees and boards. You name it, I could do it—or at least I thought I could. In the process, I lost any sense of calling, vocation, or passion. I lived out the various scripts handed to me, never stopping to ask if I was the best fit for the role. I lived with constant guilt because I could not satisfy all the expectations placed on me. It seemed I was always letting someone down.

When I began to listen to my inner voice, I found out that I was tired of being part of other people's visions, writing chapters in the books of others, and making sure their programs functioned well. There was simply no energy left to live out a passion or a vision. To find renewed passion and energy, I had to strip down. Stripping down meant asking the hard questions regarding why I reacted to others the way I did. It meant beginning to say no to requests. It meant giving myself permission to live with the disappointment and disapproval of others. It meant letting go of people who weighed me down beyond my capacity to carry them.

When I first began the process of stripping down, I faced the constant temptation to return to the well-established pattern of people pleasing. After all, it represented a way of life I had known for many decades. It was my default mode and a comfort zone of sorts. There was constant battle with my old companion—guilt. Most of all, there was the tyranny of "they." "What will they think of me?" was the question that came to my mind after saying no. "They" are powerful in the lives of women. "They" rule over us. "They" live in our psyches. "They" define us to the degree that we cannot locate our true selves without great effort.

Lynne Hybels writes about her experience of letting go of a life characterized by the desire to please others. "You can only work hard and seek love for so long. Eventually you just run out of energy. And, I did," notes Hybels.[5] Hybels lived well into her

185

forties with the driving desire to please others, to the point that she didn't know her true self. After seeking help from a therapist, she came to differentiate between the voices of others and the voice of her authentic self.

Hybels also learned to differentiate between being a girl and being a woman: "Whereas a girl of any age lives out the script she learned as a child—a script too often grounded in powerlessness—a woman acknowledges and accepts her power to change, and grow, and be a force for good in the world."[6] The transition from a girl to a woman is hard work. It requires that we let go of the script of powerlessness to become a woman garnished with power and strength from her inner being. It is to live with purpose that is self-directed. It is to have a vision.

Finding our passion involves acknowledging those things that are not truly ours and letting them go. It means listening to the inner voice speaking truth about ourselves. For me, that voice first spoke truth about the things that did not matter. It was a voice that helped me shed a life I didn't own.

Sometime later, after I cleared out the clutter of a very busy life, my heart began to speak new words. Four simple yet profoundly deep messages began to emerge: "I love the world of nature." "I love to write." "I love to preach." "I love to play with my grandchildren." Deep down I knew that I received these four messages as guiding images for the second half of my life. I am still discovering how to live them out, but I am well into this journey of discovery.

"I love the world of nature" was a message that tapped into my childhood. I grew up in the country and spent most of my time outdoors. My happiest memories are of times of imaginative play in the woods, splashing in the creek, and lying on my back in an open field, hidden from everyone by the tall grass. The sounds of nature—crickets on a summer night, the call of a bobwhite quail during a hot summer day—remain embedded deep within my psyche.

Loving nature has now become a passion and a vision. For me, that means I work toward the care of creation, which is now seriously endangered by global climate change and the ravages of modern progress. The effort to work for creation's care has meant that I write and speak about the issue. Creation is my calling. It is my passion.

"I love to write." As an academic, writing is part of my job description. In higher education, there is the dictum "Publish or perish." For this reason, being published in journals and writing monographs have been part of my existence for decades. Due to my tendency to please others, I have written too many articles out of duty and not enough out of passion. This tendency made it easy for me to agree to participate in writing projects that were not my own. For many years, I neglected writing about things that really mattered to me so that the commitments that were important to others might be fulfilled.

During the roughest part of perimenopause, I lost all energy to write. I missed deadlines and failed to keep commitments. I managed to write a few articles, but for the most part, my writing life was barren and listless. I cared little about publishing yet one more article or delivering one more academic paper at a conference.

Coming out on the other side of the menopausal journey, after acknowledging what I did not like to write, I discovered a renewed passion for writing, only now I write my own words. *Seven Transforming Gifts of Menopause* is the fruit of listening to my inner voice and embarking on a quest to write about the things that really matter to me.

"I love to preach." Acknowledging these words has been hard. I married into a religious tradition that affirms women but at the same time is highly patriarchal. This double message is difficult to live with. It means that those of us in my tradition who call ourselves ministers must pay homage to the culture of male superiority while simultaneously living out our calling. It causes us to lead a double life, having an ever-cautious awareness of the boundaries while at the same time attempting to fulfill a larger vocation that pushes against those boundaries.

I preached my first sermon at the age of sixteen. Standing before a congregation and speaking sacred, life-giving words was a wonderful experience. However, as the years passed, I moved comfortably into the academic world. Teaching religion was somewhat safer than preaching religion. During the decades of my academic career, I had opportunities to preach. I have preached around the world. One summer I served as preacher/chaplain at the Chautauqua Institution in New York. Preaching in Chautauqua's historic open-air pavilion, a place where US presidents have delivered important speeches, was a highlight of my life.

Despite the occasional opportunity, preaching was secondary to my life as a teacher. It was easier that way. It was less controversial and less threatening to men. I love to teach, but as I face the second half of my life, it no longer brings me the joy it once did. When I gave myself permission to listen to my inner, authentic self, I heard my sixteen-year-old self saying, "I love to preach." As I enter into the sixth decade of my life, I have found a new freedom to introduce myself as reverend or preacher.

"I love to play with my grandchildren." No one prepared me for the great joy of being a grandmother. Since all five of my grandchildren live out of state, it is difficult to see them. However, being with them, entering their worlds of imagination, spoiling them, and listening to them have become priorities in my life. This means I must travel more than I would like to. It means blocking out weeks during the summer in order to have them visit our farm.

I am still in the process of looking inward for my passion, for the sweet spot of living out a vision, but I am further along than I was a few years ago. Looking inward has been hard work. It has involved listening to my inner voice. It has meant letting go of ways of being in the world that were destructive to my inner well-being. I have had to work at carving out space and time for the things that bring me fulfillment and joy. In the words of Parker Palmer, I am continuing to "recover and reclaim the gift . . . once possessed."[7]

Look Outward: See the World's Great Need

It is often difficult for women who have been focused on the tight-knit world of relationships to suddenly find their place within the larger world. Developing an awareness of the self, letting go of some of the constraints of cyclical time, and grasping hold of linear time can help them look outward toward the horizon of history. However, for many women, that larger horizon and the needs of the world can be overwhelming. There are so many options in terms of lifestyle, hobbies, activities, and volunteer opportunities. It is often easier to become passive in the face of hunger, homelessness, AIDS, poverty, wars, and human trafficking than to choose a place where we can make a difference.

Looking inward and finding our deepest passions helps us focus on those things in the outer world to which we are called. For instance, Caroline's work in a food bank began after she looked inward and found that she loves helping people in tangible ways. After looking inward, she turned her gaze outward and found the food bank. She loves the feeling of boxing up food, arranging shelves, and meeting people face-to-face. Caroline's activism is a result of her primary love for the tangible and concrete actions of giving to others.

In my own life, I looked inward and discovered a love for the world of nature. Looking outward, I saw the crisis of global climate change. Opportunities to be involved came my way, and I grasped hold of those opportunities. This meeting of my inward passion and the outer world became the sweet spot for finding my larger purpose or vision. The same can be true for you.

LISA SHARON HARPER

As Lisa Sharon Harper entered her mid-forties, she had the fulfilling position of chief church engagement officer for a respected evangelical nonprofit organization. In this job, she traveled, advocated for justice, and forged relationships with Christians of various stripes. Then came the US presidential election of 2016 and the white supremacist rally in Charlottesville. These events caused Harper to look inward. As she did, she began to hear her voice as well as the hidden voices of her ancestors. She asked some hard questions: "At what point were things 'great' for my family? When we were enslaved? When freed ancestors fought for the freedom of others? When we were removed from our indigenous lands? When the colonizing U.S. annexed Puerto Rico, my father's father's homeland? When my black Puerto Rican family moved to the U.S. and was among the first to experience white flight in the South Bronx? When my great grandmother fled north to escape the racial terror and ethnic cleansing of Jim Crow South Carolina?"[8]

Harper realized there was a huge gap between the stories told by her family and the ones being told to preserve the dominant US narrative—one that protects the supremacy of whiteness. Harper observes that the narrative gap is the gap between the "stories we tell ourselves about ourselves, how we got here, and as a result, the disparate visions of what it will take to become 'great.'"⁹ In the spring of 2017, Harper visited the Apartheid Museum in Johannesburg, South Africa. The exhibit on the nation's Truth and Reconciliation Commission rocked her. The commission had three objectives:

1. Determine who had perpetrated and been victims of human rights abuses.
2. Determine the requirements for rehabilitation and reparation.
3. Determine which human rights violators would receive amnesty.

Harper came away from the Apartheid Museum impressed with the power of narrative. She realized that separation and subjugation are maintained by the silencing of people's stories. She envisioned a process of sharing and amplification of narrative that would hold the power to weave people in the US together. She determined to create a space to help shrink the narrative gap within the US.

After returning to the US, Harper transitioned out of her secure job and stepped out in faith to create Freedom Road Consulting Group. Its goals are simple: "to design conversations and experiences that bring common understanding, common commitment, and lead to common action toward a more just world."¹⁰

Today, Harper offers training to help organizations and communities understand implicit and explicit racial bias and their impact on systems, structures, and policies. She organizes forums where people from various walks of life can engage one another toward a common understanding of justice.

One of the most innovative aspects of Harper's work is her emphasis on pilgrimage. Freedom Road Pilgrimages guides groups on a multiday journey through various sites where the stories of colonization and domination occurred. At these sites, Harper leads participants in the process of listening deeply to narratives of those who suffered there.

She invites theological exploration of the concept of shalom and asks participants to carry the stories back into their communities.

Overcoming Your Fears

Women like Lisa Sharon Harper are discovering a calling to be proactive in the world, and they are not alone. Millions of women are facing the second half of their lives—women who are courageous and proactive. Imagine the energy, resources, and time that can be harnessed for good in the world when women live out of a deep inner passion. We can be world changers.

The second half of life is an opportunity to move out of the relational web and into a larger horizon of the world. "The world" can be your neighborhood, your church, or your city. It can be a faraway place where there is poverty, disease, and war. Know that there is a spot out there for you. There is a wider space into which you can move. But before you can move into that larger space, you will need to face your fears.

Fear is a powerful force. Surrendering to its power will paralyze you, making you unable to live in the beautiful space of the vision for the second half of your life. Facing and overcoming your fears will thrust you into being the woman you are meant to be.

When Lisa Sharon Harper was dreaming of stepping out in faith to launch Freedom Road, she attended a meeting where she met a woman bishop. The bishop looked at Harper and said, "I have a word from God for you. The word from the Lord for you is 'Jump!'" Harper knew instantly what the word meant. She was to step out in faith and launch the new ministry she carried in her heart. God would be there to catch her. Then in the next breath the bishop said, "I have a follow-up word: God says, 'I cannot catch you until you jump!'"[11]

192

Harper had fear about her financial future. She had fear about failure. But she also had faith that God would be there to catch her. She summoned her courage and jumped.

Take heart, fearful one. The last gift, the gift of courage, awaits you.

Personal Reflection Activities

1. As you assess your present circumstances, how are you in need of the gift of vision?
2. Describe how your menopausal self is "crying for a dream."
3. How might you find time to get away and embark on your own vision quest? Where in your area can you spend some time alone?
4. In listening to your inner voice, what is being said?

   What do you no longer want to do?

   What is your energy level?

   What no longer brings you joy?

   What things need to be released?

   What are your deep passions?

   Are you able to serve these passions?

5. In looking outward, what is calling to you?

   What brings you fulfillment?

   What are the pressing needs in your sphere of influence?

   Who needs your gifts?

6. What risks do you need to take in order to fulfill your newly emerging vision for the second half of life?

Group Reflection Activities

1. Take time to reflect on how postmenopausal women are making a difference in the world.
2. Talk about the things that no longer bring fulfillment.
3. Share dreams about the future. Offer no judgment on these dreams but encourage probing questions.
4. Discuss the issue of risk taking. What might hold women back from living out their visions?
5. End the discussion with reflection on what it means to live on autopilot—without vision for the second half of life. How can you avoid this way of living?

EIGHT

THE GIFT
OF COURAGE

The opposite of a nice girl is not a good woman, but a downright
dangerous woman.

— Lynne Hybels, *Nice Girls Don't Change the World*

Trouble will tame an advanced young woman, but an advanced
old woman is uncontrollable.

— Dorothy Sayers, *Clouds of Witness*

IN MIDLIFE, MY FRIEND DIANE made a dramatic career change, moving
from a good job in the district attorney's office to seminary for a
degree in counseling. She made this decision because she wanted
to proactively help young women like those she had seen come
through the legal system without support, goals, or any mental
counseling. When she was halfway through her education, Diane
was diagnosed with inoperable cancer. Day after day, I watched
her calmly continue her quest to become a counselor. There were
times I wondered why she even bothered. She had large tumors

195

growing in her body and had been told that no one lived past two years with her type of cancer. When I asked Diane about her decision to continue, she said, "God told me to 'occupy,' and I will occupy my time fulfilling my dreams."

Diane completed her course work, but her end would come a week before the date of graduation. The day of her death, the president of the seminary went to Diane's house and awarded her the MA degree. A few hours later, she passed away. Diane is the face of courage.

Courage is a virtue not just for women such as Diane who are facing extraordinary circumstances. It is a virtue for all of us who desire to live out our lives with passion and vision.

Courage is the critical element in the remaking of our lives during menopause. It makes the difference between a life characterized by a longing to fulfill a vision and a life lived with passion and vision. It is the difference between being paralyzed by fear and facing and overcoming fear. Courage takes an ordinary life and transforms it into one that is marked by extraordinary power.

Courage is the last gift of menopause. This gift is hidden in the deep cave of your psyche. It is your dragon self. It is the adventurous, questing person you may have known in the past but due to life's circumstances was banished to the land of fairy tales. Now is the time to return to the cave and find your dragon dreams.

Dragon Dreams

Recently, my daughter sent me a photo of my three-year-old granddaughter. The message accompanying the photo read, "Tegan having a princess tea party with Zeus the dragon." In this delightful photo, Tegan is sitting on a blanket in the living room wearing her favorite princess attire—a pink tutu and a tiara. Beside her, with his nose on the blanket, lies Zeus, their large mixed-breed shelter dog. Zeus and Tegan have been friends since her parents brought Tegan home from the hospital shortly after her birth.

Zeus is a hyperactive dog (part boxer terrier), and he has a bad habit of jumping on people. We were afraid that, in his excitement, Zeus would jump on Tegan's tiny body and harm her. Our fears were unfounded. From the get-go, Zeus was Tegan's companion and protector. Tegan was born in the first week of March, a time when the weather is cold in Wheaton, Illinois. During the first weeks of Tegan's life, her parents placed her on a blanket on the floor in front of a gently blowing space heater. Zeus would position himself there, partly to get the warmth but also to keep watch over Tegan. If she stirred while her parents were in another room, he would go running to them with an anxious look on his face. As Tegan grew, she and Zeus became playmates, chasing each other through the house.

Zeus is Tegan's "dragon dog." In her imagination, he is the dragon who keeps watch over her castle. From time to time, Tegan will invite Zeus to tea parties in this castle—a blanket on the floor. There Zeus takes the same position he once held when Tegan was a newborn—on the floor with his nose on the blanket. He is content to be there, and sometimes Tegan will place a cup and saucer in front of him, saying, "Here, Zeus, have some tea."

Tegan has discovered the world of princesses, castles, and dragons. She knows that dragons are powerful creatures and that sometimes they are not very nice. Whenever I visit, she will come up to me and whisper, "Nanny, there is a dragon in my room." This statement begins our dragon quest. "There is?" I reply. "Is he a good dragon?" "I don't know," answers Tegan. "Well," I say to her, "let's go in your room and see." We run to her room, where she exclaims, "There he is!" I ask the dragon, "Are you a good dragon?" Turning to Tegan, I tell her, "Yes, he says he is a good dragon and he has come to play."

Tegan has not yet learned that princesses do not play with dragons. She has not yet been given the script telling her that one day she will need a prince to slay the dragon and take her away to a place where they will live happily ever after. I wish I could keep Tegan from this narrative, but I know I cannot. Right now, her parents and I work on helping Tegan to have a healthy respect for the power of dragons but not to be afraid of them. We want her life to be filled with dragon quests.

Sara Maitland, in the short story "Dragon Dreams," masterfully rewrites the classic tale of *George and the Dragon*.[1] In Maitland's story, the princess of the tale is somewhere in midlife. Years have passed since she called George to come rescue her and slay the dragon. By this time, she has suffered the death of her only child and a divorce from her prince. Now the princess is writing to the dragon, calling for him to return to her. As the letter unfolds, the reader discovers that the princess had a relationship with the dragon long before she called for George to slay him. Their relationship was not one of animosity and fear. It was one of wonder, love, and courage. It is this relationship that she longs to restore.

Reflecting on the events that led up to George slaying the dragon, the princess writes, "All those years ago I made a terrible mistake . . . but, you frightened me." She continues, "I was afraid of the dragon of me, the great ferocious growling monster of rage and passion." The princess knew that she had the power to become a dragon woman but that if she did she "would never be ordinary ever again." She would have to go with the dragon into the hot, searing desert and live with him. The ancient dragon in her "would gobble up all the sweet little girl . . . and there would be nothing left of all my pettiness and silliness."[2]

This thought was too much for the young princess. She "suddenly wanted only to be the sort of ordinary princess who goes to the supermarket with a shopping trolley." Looking back through the years, the princess confesses to the dragon, "In a moment of weakness, I wanted an ordinary boring prince to appear on a white charger and rescue me. . . . I thought he would keep me safe from my own desires."[3]

The princess knew that the dragon let himself be killed for her. "And it nearly broke my heart." She laments, "Moral cowardice is a leprosy to the soul, it shrivels it up and makes the sinner small. So after that I just forgot the whole damn thing. . . . Lots of princesses do, we are brought up to it you know, and it is harder to change than one might think."[4]

The princess had awakened to a startling reality: "When my child died, . . . I knew there was no safety, anywhere . . . but there is wildness and joy, there is love and life within the danger." She ends her letter with a plea to the dragon: "I love you. I want to be with you. I want to reclaim my dragon soul and fly. . . . This letter is just a start. I am going to hunt you down now in all the lovely desolate places of the world. You are Questing Beast, like the valiant knights in olden days. Wherever there is a perfect sunrise, a dark cliff, a small pool of water, a distant city wreathed in morning mist, there I will be waiting for you. Please come. Please come soon."[5]

In "Dragon Dreams," Maitland has given women in midlife a map for finding the gift of courage. The letter written by the princess reveals the steps you need to take to become the dragon woman you are meant to be: (1) return to your dragon space, (2) remember your earlier dragon self, (3) reflect on how you lost the dragon, and (4) envision your future with the dragon.

How to Claim the Gift of Courage

Return to Your Dragon Space

During the time of melancholy surrounding the death of her child and her divorce, the princess returns to the place where she first met the dragon. This returning stirs up memories long repressed—memories of an earlier self and memories of a time when she was a different person. "There is something mysterious about memory," writes the princess. "Recapturing memories revives one."[6] It was these memories that led the princess to want to seek out the dragon.

At midlife, it is important for us women to remember the days when we were a much younger version of ourselves. Remembering helps revive us, breathing new life into lives that may have been put to sleep. We were the youth who dared to risk and to dream. We were the girls who played with gusto, danced with energy, and loved with passion. We did not know the restraints of aging and responsibilities. We did not know the disappointments of betrayed relationships that would leave us alone and afraid. We were once dragon girls.

In returning to the space where our spirits were free, we call to the dragon girl who still lives in the caves of our psyches. We can stand where she stood. We can dance where she danced. We can dream where she dreamed.

My dragon space is the town of Wheaton, Illinois. It is where my husband and I moved two weeks after our wedding. We arrived the first of January in 1975 with no money and no promise of jobs. We had acceptance into graduate school and a place to live. We had our faith in a God who had called us out of our native southern soil to the Chicago area. Somehow those things were enough.

My daughter now lives in this town, along with her husband and children. Whenever I visit, I walk the sidewalks where I once walked as a young, adventurous grad student. I take my grandchildren down the prairie path where my husband and I rode clunky bicycles that we found in the basement of the old house we were renting. I stop and stare at the ground where the old house we lived in once stood. This was a questing ground. This was my place of courage. Here was where I lived in faith and in a spirit of adventure. Here was where my husband and I kneeled beside our bed and prayed for rent money. This was the place where the exact amount of money we needed arrived in our mailbox the following morning. Wheaton is where my husband and I launched out into the deep. Returning to the place brings back the same feelings of excitement and courage.

Look for the places where you once knew the dragon. Return there and recall what it was like to be young and daring. This place may be a college campus. This place may be a foreign country where you were once an exchange student. It may be where you made your first home. It may be your home church.

If you cannot return physically to your dragon place, do so in your imagination. Recall the sights, sounds, smells, and feel of your questing place. Take time to remember what it felt like to be full of dreams. Do you recall answered prayers? Do you remember the dreams?

Remember Your Earlier Dragon Self

The princess in Maitland's story recalls the joy and thrills of knowing the dragon. She remembers being enthralled by the astonishing strength of his wings and the stunning moment when she first saw his silhouette dance against the sunset: "Had I not felt, in myself, my own magic power, my strength, that could match yours and make us a fitting couple?"[7]

The process of remembering helps revive us. We cannot go back in time, but we can reclaim what time has stripped away or buried. Recall when you took risks—riding a roller coaster, hiking the Appalachian Trail, moving to a new place to attend school, buying your first home. Maybe you were the adventurous young woman who believed the world was hers for the taking.

As you reflect on these times of adventure and risk, consider how you felt during those moments. Did you not feel your own magic power and strength? What price were you willing to pay to take the risk? Can you remember that part of your self that relished the adventure despite the possibilities of failure? Do you remember what it felt like to live with the guiding presence of the Holy Spirit? Do you remember what it was like to be so full of faith that you had no fear of what the future would bring?

My husband and I have a saying we use when we recall our younger days when we were willing to move across the country to attend graduate school without money or jobs. We often say, "We just didn't know any better." You may recall what it was like not to know any better. Now that you know better, how might you bring back some of that adventurous earlier self? In midlife, it is tempting to seek safety in retirement accounts, jobs, and homes. If we are not careful, these things can cause us to forget what it was like when we didn't know any better.

Listen to the words of the princess: "I knew there was no safety, anywhere . . . but there is wildness and joy, there is love and life within the danger."[8] In the safest of places, there is death, divorce, economic recessions, and cancer. Accepting this fact helps you not know any better than to risk adventure in the second half of life.

The young woman of your earlier life is alive within you, but you must remember her. Remember her to the degree that you can feel her energy. Remember her to the degree that your blood runs with her pulse. She will help you find a new passion and excitement for today's challenges and decisions. She will take you by the hand and lead you into a future where there is no safety but wildness and joy in the danger.

Reflect On How You Lost the Dragon

Perhaps the hardest part of finding your courage is remembering how you lost it in the first place. We do not suddenly become people who settle for the ordinary and the safe places. Such things happen to us in increments of time as we bargain away our questing selves for the promises of security.

The princess in Maitland's story was affected by the pull of the safe realm of the ordinary world of shopping carts and the security of "an ordinary boring prince ... [who would] rescue me." Furthermore, the princess knew that she was not alone in her choice to call for George to slay the dragon. In her letter, the princess lets the dragon know that she was not the only one who was afraid of the dragon woman. Her mother and father and all those around her wanted her to be "their sweet virgin princess." They did not want her to be a fierce dragon woman, although, as she writes, "It was my truth."9

The princess's choice of the safe route was in keeping with the expectations of her family and the world in which she lived. Young women are encouraged to become princesses. They are encouraged to seek the roads of safety found in the myth of a rescuing man. Marriage does not always imply such a tale, but it often does. Too often marriage requires a woman to give up her truth in order to fit into the life of another. Rare are the marriages that offer the route of a joint quest or a joint adventure.

If your marriage is one that called you to leave behind your questing self, menopause is the time to revisit the purpose of your partnership. It is a good time to talk openly and freely with your husband regarding your sense of loss. Open talk helps to heal the wounds. If you keep things hidden in the recesses of your psyche, you cannot claim the gift of courage. Hiding is the coward's route.

If you are married, the best and healthiest way for you to receive the gift of courage is for you and your partner to revisit the conditions of your marriage and to analyze together how you both took the roads of safety, playing the scripted roles of marriage. Perhaps your husband did not actually want an ordinary princess. Maybe, just maybe, he wanted a dragon woman for a questing partner in the grand adventure of life.

From time to time, a male student will approach me after class with the question, "Dr. Johns, how can I help my wife not to be so passive? I love her supporting me in my career, but it seems that when I ask her about her life, she draws a blank." One young man actually complained that his wife "just wants to do what I want her to do." He told me, "I am so tired of directing her life."

If you have not already done so, join your spouse in seeking the lands of adventure. Menopause can be the time when you become each other's questing partner. The transition from a traditional marriage to one characterized by authentic partnership will not be easy for either of you. But if you go forward together, with love and mutual respect, you can find a dimension of being together that is much deeper and more exciting than what you had before.

In your own journey toward your questing self, you may encounter resistance from your spouse to your new way of being in the world. You can honor the covenant of marriage while at the same time reclaiming your dragon self. Honoring a marriage covenant is not the same as keeping things the same. Marriage is deeper than prescribed roles. It is a bond that goes deeper than contractual agreements. The marriage covenant is designed to survive all seasons of life, including menopause.

I will be honest with you. During my menopausal transformation, my husband and I experienced some rough patches. Both of us had settled into routines and prescribed roles. Some of those were healthy; some were not. We had to sort through things. Most of all, we had to remember. We had to remember the adventurous young couple who encouraged each other to take risks, color outside the lines, and follow God's leading.

Know that you have within you the courage to forge ahead into the place of your dragon self. You are no longer sleeping. Awakened women can go back to the way things were, but they do so at the risk of denying their truth. Truth denied is still truth. Denying it will not make it go away.

Women who are divorced or widowed have their own journey toward reclaiming their courageous selves. It may be that they abandoned their dragon selves in the pain of loss. The void of abandonment and loss can become the ground for a new life. Women in this space face the choice of retreating into pain or being reborn in the crucible of pain. Waneda's reclamation of her earlier, adventurous self came from the ruins of her husband's death and her experience with breast cancer. Her dream took her back to her childhood home. She remembered what it was like to be fifteen and filled with possibilities. She took hold of her earlier dragon self, and the world became her questing ground.

Singleness also provides a unique opportunity to become a dragon woman. When Margaret Gaines was nineteen, she boarded a steamer ship to Tunisia. Her quest was to show God's love to the Arabs.[10] Years later, Margaret settled in the village of Aboud, on the West Bank of Israel. Aboud became her home, and the Palestinian people became her family. She built a church and established a school for the village children.

Over the decades, Margaret became known as the village's "holy woman." During times of war, people would crowd into her small home, believing her presence would protect them from harm. Whenever Margaret drove through the crowded streets of Aboud, shopkeepers would stop what they were doing in order to motion for cars and pedestrians to make way for her small VW Beetle.

Whenever I had the privilege of being in Margaret's presence, who I often referred to as Saint Margaret, I was in awe of her strength. She frightened me, but at the same time I was drawn to the spiritual energy that radiated from her. Margaret would often tell me, "I see people bound to their possessions. I possess little, so my energy is focused on serving the Palestinian people." Margaret Gaines could never be described as a "nice woman." She lived beyond the world of living up to the expectations of others. She was a fierce dragon woman.

Whether we are married or single, each of us carries within us a memory of an earlier time when we played in the dragon's den. Many of us have a memory of calling for the dragon slayer and taking the safe route. Yet all of us have the potential to reclaim our status as dragon women.

Envision Your Future with the Dragon

The princess not only remembers her life with the dragon but also envisions herself with him again. "I love you," she writes. "I want to be with you. I want to reclaim my dragon soul and fly. I refuse to believe we only get one chance. . . . I am going to hunt you down now in all the lovely desolate places of the world."[11] Desire is a strong motivator. It can be a catalyst for courage. Desire can pull us out of a safe and secure place and thrust us into an uncharted land. If we desire that noble and adventurous part of ourselves to return, we can call her out and reclaim her. Can you say with the princess, "I want to reclaim my dragon soul and fly"? If so, you are well on your journey toward claiming the gift of courage.

You may ask, "What about the fear I feel?" Courage is not the absence of fear. It is deciding not to allow the fear to keep you from living a full life. Refuse to believe you get only one chance in life to fulfill your dreams. Refuse to believe that the past is a certain predictor of the future. Call to your dragon, and reclaim your dragon soul.

Community of the Courageous

In 2003, thousands of women living amid the violence of civil war in Liberia united for the cause of peace in their country. After years of suffering under the brutal rule of Charles Taylor and watching their sons die in the senseless violence of civil war, Liberia's women had had enough. The movement, organized by social worker Leymah Gbowee, began small—with praying and singing in a fish market. But it quickly spread as thousands of women joined together in an effort to "pray the devil back to hell."[12]

Armed with only white T-shirts and the courage born of a desire for peace, the "white army" of women marched, pressured leaders to hold peace talks, and staged protests in front of the palace of the president. As a result of their efforts, Liberia saw the end of a fourteen-year-long civil war and the election of Liberia's first woman president, Ellen Johnson Sirleaf.

Leymah Gbowee did not bring an end to Liberia's civil war by working as a solitary hero. She called upon her community of sisters. Together, they did what no conventional armies could do. Kathleen Fischer writes, "Courage is not a quality of the solitary self. It is created and sustained in community. Even when alone, we draw on others to strengthen us. Courage is born in the experience of being loved and upheld. It is rooted in grace."[13]

The force of women's corporate courage is on the rise. Together, we are daring to pray the devil back to hell. We are pushing back the darkness of sexism and its powerful offspring—misogyny. We are finding our courageous voices; together, we sing, preach, and write. We are putting our words into action by marching, running for political office, and standing behind pulpits. We are organizing against human trafficking and child abuse. We are organizing on behalf of refugees and the working poor. We are women of valor.

Personal Reflection Activities

1. Describe your dragon self. How has this part of you been lost through the years?
2. Reflect on how life experiences have chipped away at your courage. What are your current fears?
3. Describe your dragon space. What was it like to live there?
4. Write your own letter to the dragon.

   What would you say about your past?
   What caused you to banish the dragon?
   If the dragon returns, what would your life look like?
   Describe your dragon-questing self.

5. If you are married, how can you join with your spouse in living a more adventurous life?
6. How can you become part of a larger community of courageous women?

Group Reflection Activities

1. Take a few minutes to review the section "Dragon Dreams." Reflect on how you may or may not identify with the princess in the story.
2. Open the floor to anyone who would like to share about their earlier dragon self. Reflect on the images and memories shared.
3. Discuss the ways women lose their courage. What life events contribute to this loss? What does a life look like without courage?
4. Discuss this sentence: "I knew there was no safety, anywhere . . . but there is wildness and joy, there is love and life within the danger." How does God's presence within the danger make a difference?
5. Envision a life with courage. Share with one another what needs to change in order for you to live this life.
6. End with a blessing.

As you travel through the land of menopause, may you claim its gifts:

the gift of uncovering
the gift of anger
the gift of the authentic self
the gift of expanded time
the gift of spiritual freedom
the gift of vision
the gift of courage

May all of these gifts come together in the place where you claim your courageous dragon soul and fly!

NOTES

Introduction

1. Pat Wingert and Barbara Kantrowitz, *The Menopause Book* (New York: Workman Publishing, 2009), 13.

2. Wingert and Kantrowitz, *The Menopause Book*, 13.

3. "Estrogen Deficiency States," Cleveland Clinic, https://my.cleveland clinic.org/health/diseases/16978-estrogen-deficiency-states.

4. "Depression at Perimenopause: More than Just Hormones," Harvard Health Publishing, August 2008, http://www.health.harvard.edu/womens -health/depression-at-perimenopause.

5. Christiane Northrup, *The Wisdom of Menopause: Creating Physical and Emotional Health during the Change* (New York: Bantam Books, 2001), 120.

6. Wingert and Kantrowitz, *Menopause Book*, 18–19.

7. Quoted in Louise Foxcroft, *Hot Flushes, Cold Science: A History of the Modern Menopause* (Granta, UK: Granta Books, 2010), 81.

8. Foxcroft, *Hot Flushes, Cold Science*, 120.

9. Foxcroft, *Hot Flushes, Cold Science*, 125.

10. "Female Hysteria during Victorian Era: Its Symptoms, Diagnosis, Treatment/Cures," http://victorian-era.org/female-hysteria-during-victorian -era.html.

11. "Female Hysteria during Victorian Era."

12. Laura Briggs, "The Race of Hysteria: 'Overcivilization' and the 'Savage' Woman in Late Nineteenth Century Obstetrics and Gynecology, *American Quarterly* 52, no. 2 (2000): 246–73.

13. Foxcroft, *Hot Flushes, Cold Science*, 142.

14. Quoted in Foxcroft, *Hot Flushes, Cold Science*, 135.

15. Robert Kistner, "Gynecology: Durable, Unendurable Women," *Time,* October 16, 1964, 72.

16. Robert Wilson, *Feminine Forever* (New York: Pocket Books, 1968). As late as 2018, Wilson's book still garnered five-star ratings on Amazon.

17. Robert Wilson, "The Fate of the Nontreated Postmenopausal Woman: A Plea for the Maintenance of Adequate Estrogen from Puberty to the Grave," *Journal of the American Geriatric Society* 11, no. 4 (1963): 347–62.

18. "Estrogen and Hormones," The Cleveland Clinic, April 29, 2019, https://my.clevelandclinic.org/health/articles/16979-estrogen-hormones.

19. Gail Sheehy, *Menopause: The Silent Passage* (New York: Random House, 1991).

20. Sheehy, *Menopause,* 60.

21. Sheehy, *Menopause,* xix.

22. See note 5 (above) for the full citation.

23. James Loder, *The Transforming Moment,* 2nd ed. (Colorado Springs: Helmers & Howard, 1989).

24. Loder, *Transforming Moment,* 90.

25. Sue Monk Kidd, *When the Heart Waits: Spiritual Direction for Life's Sacred Questions* (New York: HarperOne, 1990), 83.

Chapter 1 Puberty and the Relational Self

1. Mary Pipher, *Reviving Ophelia: Saving the Selves of Adolescent Girls* (New York: Putnam, 1994), 39.

2. Bruno Bettelheim, *The Uses of Enchantment* (New York: Knopf, 1976), 225–36.

3. Pipher, *Reviving Opheila,* 19.

4. Carol Gilligan, *In a Different Voice* (Cambridge, MA: Harvard University Press, 1982).

5. Christiane Northrup, *The Wisdom of Menopause: Creating Physical and Emotional Health during the Change* (New York: Bantam Books, 2001), 51.

6. Northrup, *Wisdom of Menopause,* 51.

7. Jean Baker Miller, *Toward a New Psychology of Women* (Boston: Beacon Press, 1976), 83.

Chapter 2 The Gift of Uncovering

1. Richard Rohr, *Falling Upward: A Spirituality for the Two Halves of Life* (San Francisco: Jossey-Bass, 2011), vii.

2. Christiane Northrup, *The Wisdom of Menopause: Creating Physical and Emotional Health during the Change* (New York: Bantam Books, 2001), 41.

3. For a more detailed description of the hormonal shifts and their effect on the brain, see Christiane Northrup, "The Brain Catches Fire at Menopause," in *Wisdom of Menopause*, 36–75.

4. Northrup, *Wisdom of Menopause*, 55.

5. Northrup, *Wisdom of Menopause*, 42.

6. Sue Monk Kidd, *When the Heart Waits* (New York: HarperOne, 1990), 91.

7. Kidd, *When the Heart Waits*, 101.

8. Northrup, *Wisdom of Menopause*, 150.

9. Carolyn Scott Brown, with Barbara S. Levy, *The Black Woman's Guide to Menopause: Doing Menopause with Heart and Soul* (Naperville, IL: Source-Books, 2003), 21.

10. Jonathan Martin, *How to Survive a Shipwreck: Help Is on the Way and Love Is Already Here* (Grand Rapids: Zondervan, 2016), 24.

11. Northrup, *Wisdom of Menopause*, 17.

12. Quoted in Kidd, *When the Heart Waits*, 92.

13. Louise Foxcroft, *Hot Flushes, Cold Science: A History of the Modern Menopause* (Granta, UK: Granta Books, 2010), 50.

14. Quoted in Foxcroft, *Hot Flushes, Cold Science*, 68.

15. Northrup, *Wisdom of Menopause*, 269.

16. S. Shanmugan, T. D. Satterthwaite, M. D. Sammel, et al. "Impact of Early Life Adversity and Tryptophan Depletion on Functional Connectivity in Menopausal Women," *Psychoneuroendocrinology* 84 (2017): 197–205.

17. Michael Tannenbaum, "Penn Study Finds Teen Trauma Causes Depression Risk in Menopause," *Philly Voice*, March 29, 2017, https://www.phillyvoice.com/penn-study-finds-teen-trauma-raises-depression-risk-menopause.

18. Elaine Johnson, "Black Women Endure Menopause Longest," *San Diego Voice and Viewpoint*, February 25, 2015.

19. Audre Lorde, *Sister Outsider* (Berkeley, CA: Crossing Press, 2007), 117.

20. Interview with Lisa Sharon Harper, May 5, 2019.

21. Lisa Sharon Harper, "This Is the Cost of Our History," *Sojourners*, May 2019, https://sojo.net/magazine/may-2019/cost-our-history.

22. Dan Hurley, "Grandma's Experiences Leave a Mark on Your Genes," *Discover*, May 2013, http://www.discovermagazine.com/2013/may/13-grandmas-experiences-leave-epigenetic-mark-on-your-genes.

Chapter 3 The Gift of Anger

1. Christiane Northrup, *The Wisdom of Menopause* (New York: Bantam Books, 2001), 54.

2. Soraya Chemaly, *Rage Becomes Her: The Power of Women's Anger* (New York: Simon & Schuster, 2018), 261.

3. Harriet Lerner, *The Dance of Anger: A Women's Guide to Changing the Patterns of Intimate Relationships* (New York: HarperCollins, 2005), 3.

4. Christiane Northrup, *The Secret Pleasures of Menopause* (Carlsbad, CA: Hay House, 2008), 7.

5. Chemaly, *Rage Becomes Her*, 295.

6. Lerner, *Dance of Anger*, 5.

7. Lerner, *Dance of Anger*, 5.

8. Northrup, *Wisdom of Menopause*, 57.

9. Northrup, *Wisdom of Menopause*, 58–59.

10. Northrup, *Wisdom of Menopause*, 59.

11. Heather Sells, "#ChurchToo Movement about to Take Off?," CBN News, February 6, 2018, https://www1.cbn.com/cbnnews/us/2018/february/churchtoo-movement-about-to-take-off.

12. Heather Sells, "Max Lucado Reveals His Sexual Abuse, Beth Moore Challenges Churches at Summit," CBN News, December 14, 2018, https://www1.cbn.com/cbnnews/cwn/2018/december/max-lucado-reveals-his-sexual-abuse-beth-moore-challenges-church-at-churchtoo-summit.

13. https://#silenceisnotspiritual.org.

14. Quoted in Elizabeth Johnson, *She Who Is: The Mystery of God in Feminist Theological Discourse* (New York: Herder & Herder, 2008), 85.

15. Johnson, *She Who Is*, 86.

16. Audre Lorde, *Sister Outsider* (Berkeley, CA: Crossing Press, 2007), 127.

17. Austin Channing Brown, *I'm Still Here: Black Dignity in a World Made for Whiteness* (New York: Convergent Books, 2018).

18. Brown, *I'm Still Here*, 124.

19. Brown, *I'm Still Here*, 126.

20. Chemaly, *Rage Becomes Her*, 263.

21. Chemaly, *Rage Becomes Her*, 262.

22. Chemaly, *Rage Becomes Her*, 264.

23. Chemaly, *Rage Becomes Her*, 264–65.

24. Chemaly, *Rage Becomes Her*, 265.

25. Northrup, *Secret Pleasures of Menopause*, 7.

Chapter 4 The Gift of the Authentic Self

1. Harriet Lerner, *The Dance of Anger: A Women's Guide to Changing the Patterns of Intimate Relationships* (New York: HarperCollins, 2005), 30.

2. Lerner, *Dance of Anger*, 30.

3. Marian Van Eyk McCain, *Transformation through Menopause* (New York: Bergin & Garvey, 1991), 104.

4. Kim Shaw, "God's Grace in Menopause," CBMW.org, September 4, 2013, https://cbmw.org/topics/womanhood-blog/gods-grace-in-menopause/.

5. McCain, *Transformation through Menopause*, 103.

6. Brené Brown, *The Gifts of Imperfection* (Center City, MN: Hazeldon Publishing, 2010), 50.

7. Brown, *Gifts of Imperfection*, 51.

8. Brown, *Gifts of Imperfection*, 51.

9. McCain, *Transformation through Menopause*, 105.

10. Lynne Hybels, *Nice Girls Don't Change the World* (Grand Rapids: Zondervan, 2005), 32.

11. Hybels, *Nice Girls Don't Change the World*, 35.

12. Hybels, *Nice Girls Don't Change the World*, 89.

13. See Richard Louv, *Last Child in the Woods: Saving Our Children from Nature-Deficit Disorder* (Chapel Hill: Algonquin Books, 2008).

14. "Vitamin D Deficiency Bad for the Heart, Bones, and Rest of the Body," December 2009, https://www.health.harvard.edu/press_releases/vitamin-d -deficiency-bad-for-the-heart-bones-and-rest-of-the-body.

15. Copyright © 1998 by Wendell Berry, "The Peace of Wild Things," from *The Selected Poems of Wendell Berry*. Reprinted by permission of Counterpoint Press.

16. Gregory N. Bratman, J. Paul Hamilton, Kevin S. Hahn, et al., "Nature Experience Reduces Rumination and Subgenual Prefrontal Cortex Activation," *Proceedings of the National Academy of the Sciences of the United States of America*, July 14, 2015, https://www.pnas.org/content/112/28/8567.

17. Harriet Sherwood, "Getting Back to Nature: How Forest Bathing Can Make Us Feel Better," *The Guardian*, June 8, 2019, https://www.theguardian .com/environment/2019/jun/08/forest-bathing-japanese-practice-in-west -wellbeing.

18. Allison Aubrey, "Forest Bathing: A Retreat to Nature Can Boost Immunity and Mood," NPR, July 17, 2017, https://www.npr.org/sections/health -shots/2017/07/17/536676954/forest-bathing-a-retreat-to-nature-can -boost-immunity-and-mood.

19. Brown, *Gifts of Imperfection*, 16.

20. Emerson Eggerichs, *Love and Respect* (Nashville: Thomas Nelson, 2004), 15.

21. Leonard Sax, *Girls on the Edge: The Four Factors Driving the Crisis for Girls—Sexual Identity, CyberBubble, Obsessions, Environmental Toxins* (New York: Basic Books, 2010), 75.

22. https://peacefulwife.com.

23. Sue Monk Kidd, *When the Heart Waits: Spiritual Direction for Life's Sacred Questions* (New York: HarperOne, 1990), 161.

Chapter 5 The Gift of Expanded Time

1. Tom Brokaw, *The Greatest Generation* (New York: Random House, 2005), 142.

2. Robert Wilson, "Hormone Therapy Aid to Vitality," *Los Angeles Times*, August 2, 1966, section C, 4.

3. Robert Wilson, "Love Fulfillment Helpful," *Los Angeles Times*, August 2, 1966, section H, 15.

4. Gail Sheehy, *Menopause: The Silent Passsage* (New York, Random House, 1991), 62.

5. Sue Monk Kidd, *When the Heart Waits* (New York: HarperOne, 1990), 105.

6. Kidd, *When the Heart Waits*, 105.

7. Jay Griffiths, *A Sideways Look at Time* (New York: Penguin Books, 2002), 145.

8. Quoted in Louise Foxcroft, *Hot Flushes, Cold Science: A History of the Modern Menopause* (Granta, UK: Granta Books, 2010), 61.

9. For information on endocrine disrupting chemicals, see https://www.endocrine.org.

10. Study published in PLoS One, January 2015, https://journals.plos.org/plosone/article?id=10.1371/journal.pone.0116057.

11. "Relieve Adrenal Fatigue by Normalizing Cortisol Levels," Women's Health Network, https://www.womenshealthnetwork.com/adrenal-fatigue-and-stress/relieve-adrenal-fatigue-by-normalizing-high-cortisol.aspx.

12. "Repaying Your Sleep Debt," Harvard Women's Health Watch, May 9, 2018, https://www.health.harvard.edu/womens-health/repaying-your-sleep-debt.

13. Simone de Beauvoir, *The Second Sex*, trans. H. M. Parshley (New York: Alfred Knopf, 1971), chap. 20.

14. Quoted in Sylvie de Toledo and Deborah Edler Brown, *Grandparents as Parents: A Survival Guide for Raising a Second Family*, 2nd ed. (New York: Guilford Press, 2013), 11.

15. Griffiths, *Sideways Look at Time*, 138.

16. Sara Tatyana Bernstein, "Menocore Is as Much about Wealth as It Is about Age," *Racked*, October 18, 2017, https://www.racked.com/2017/10/18/16453412/menocore-wealth-age-eileen-fisher.

17. Carl Jung, *Modern Man in Search of a Soul*, trans. W. S. Dell and Cary F. Baynes (New York: Harcourt, 1955), 58.

Chapter 6 The Gift of Spiritual Freedom

1. Sue Monk Kidd, *When the Heart Waits* (New York: HarperOne, 1990), 152.

2. Richard Rohr, *Falling Upward: A Spirituality for the Two Halves of Life* (San Francisco: Jossey-Bass, 2011), 7.

3. Carol Gilligan, "Teaching Shakespeare's Sister: Notes from the Underground in Female Adolescence," in *Making Connections: The Relational World of Adolescent Girls at Emma Willard School*, ed. Carol Gilligan, Nono Lyons, and Trudy J. Hanmer (Cambridge, MA: Harvard University Press, 1990), 6–27.

4. Patricia Davis, *Beyond Nice: The Spiritual Wisdom of Adolescent Girls* (Minneapolis: Fortress, 2001), 27.

5. Carl Jung, "The State of Psychotherapy Today," in *The Collected Works of Carl Jung*, ed. Gerhard Adler (Princeton University Press, 1970), 10:345.

6. Beth Moore, "A Letter to My Brothers," The LPM Blog, May 3, 2018, https://blog.lproof.org/2018/05/a-letter-to-my-brothers.html.

7. Rohr, *Falling Upward*, 27.

8. William Martin, *A Prophet with Honor: The Billy Graham Story*, updated ed. (Grand Rapids: Zondervan, 2018).

9. Quoted in Donald Dayton and Douglas Strong, *Rediscovering an Evangelical Heritage: A Tradition and Trajectory of Integrating Piety and Justice*, 2nd ed. (Grand Rapids: Baker Academic, 2014), 136.

10. Judith Bennett gives three main meanings of the word *patriarchy*: (1) male ecclesiastical leaders, such as the patriarch in Greek Orthodoxy; (2) legal power of male household heads (fathers/husbands); and (3) a society that promotes male privilege. Judith Bennett, *History Matters: Patriarchy and the Challenge of Feminism* (Philadelphia: University of Pennsylvania Press, 2006), 55, quoted in Beth Allison Barr, "Disrupting Christian Patriarchy: Russell Moore Is Right (Sort of)," February 20, 2019, https://www.patheos.com/blogs/anxiousbench /2019/02/disrupting-christian-patriarchy-russell-moore-is-right.

11. Carolyn Custis James, *Malestrom: Manhood Swept into the Currents of a Changing World* (Grand Rapids: Zondervan, 2015).

12. Interview with Sarah Schneiders, "God Is More Than Two Men and a Bird," *U.S. Catholic* 55, no. 5 (May 1990): 24.

13. Jackie David Johns, "The Holy Spirit: He Is a She, or Not," Jackie Speaks, November 8, 2012, https://jackiespeaks.blogspot.com/search?q=holy+spirit.

14. See Johns, "Holy Spirit."

15. Sebastian Brock, *Fire from Heaven: Studies in Syriac Theology and Liturgy* (Burlington, VT: Ashgate, 2006), 252.

16. Johns, "Holy Spirit."

17. The term *Being in Communion* is foundational for the theology of Greek Orthodoxy. See John Zizioulas, *Being as Communion* (Yonkers, NY: St. Vladimir's Seminary Press, 1997).

18. Elizabeth Johnson, *She Who Is: The Mystery of God in Feminist Theological Discourse* (New York: Herder & Herder, 2008), 222.

19. Ann Bedford Ulanov, *Finding Space: Winnicott, God, and Psychic Reality* (Louisville, KY: Westminster John Knox, 2007), 78.

20. Clement of Alexandria, *The Sacred Writings of Clement of Alexandria* §37, in Ante-Nicene Fathers, trans. Philip Schaff (Altenmünster, Germany: Jazzybee Verlag, 2017), 2:316.

21. Ulanov, *Finding Space*, 70.

22. See Jean Piaget, *The Psychology of the Child* (New York: Basic Books, 2000).

23. Quoted in Rosemary Agonito, *History of Ideas on Women: A Source Book* (New York: Parragon Books, 1977), 131.

24. "The Condition of Education: College Enrollment Rates," National Center for Education Statistics, February 2019, https://nces.ed.gov/programs /coe/indicator_cpb.asp.

25. Martin Luther King Jr., *Strength to Love* (Minneapolis: Fortress, 2010), 1.

Chapter 7 The Gift of Vision

1. Dale Hanson Bourke, *Embracing Your Second Calling: Finding Passion and Purpose for the Rest of Your Life* (Nashville: Thomas Nelson, 2009), 187.

2. Bourke, *Embracing Your Second Calling*, 107.

3. Frederick Buechner, *Wishful Thinking: A Theological ABC* (New York: Harper & Row, 1993), 95.

4. Parker Palmer, *Let Your Life Speak: Listening for the Voice of Vocation* (San Francisco: Jossey-Bass, 2000),12.

5. Lynn Hybels, *Nice Girls Don't Change the World* (Grand Rapids: Zondervan, 2005), 19.

6. Hybels, *Nice Girls Don't Change the World*, 23.

7. Palmer, *Let Your Life Speak*, 12.

8. Lisa Sharon Harper, "Let's Meet on Freedom Road," Freedom Road, November 8, 2017, https://freedomroad.us/2017/11/lets-meet-on-freedom -road.

9. Harper, "Let's Meet on Freedom Road."

10. Harper, "Let's Meet on Freedom Road."

11. Interview with Lisa Sharon Harper, May 21, 2019.

Chapter 8 The Gift of Courage

1. Sara Maitland, "Dragon Dreams," in *Angel Maker: The Short Stories of Sara Maitland* (New York: Henry Holt Books, 1996).

2. Maitland, "Dragon Dreams," 308.

3. Maitland, "Dragon Dreams," 309.

4. Maitland, "Dragon Dreams," 309.

5. Maitland, "Dragon Dreams," 309.

6. Maitland, "Dragon Dreams," 306.

7. Maitland, "Dragon Dreams," 307.

8. Maitland, "Dragon Dreams," 309.

9. Maitland, "Dragon Dreams," 308.

10. For more on Margaret Gaines's life story, see her autobiography, *Of Like Passions: Missionary to the Arabs* (Cleveland, TN: Pathway Press, 2000).

11. Maitland, "Dragon Dreams," 309.

12. The documentary *Pray the Devil Back to Hell* provides a powerful glimpse into the efforts of Liberia's women to restore peace to their country.

13. Kathleen Fischer, *Autumn Gospel: Women in the Second Half of Life* (Mahwah, NJ: Paulist Press, 1997), 37.

INDEX

221